DIFFERENTIAL DIAGNOSIS OF NEUROMUSCULOSKELETAL DISORDERS

LAWRENCE H. WYATT, DC, DACBR
Associate Professor, Division of Clinics
Dean of Clinics
Texas Chiropractic College
Pasadena, Texas

AN ASPEN PUBLICATION®
Aspen Publishers, Inc.
Gaithersburg, Maryland
1994

Library of Congress Cataloging-in-Publication Data

Wyatt, Lawrence H.
Differential diagnosis of neuromusculoskeletal disorders /
Lawrence H. Wyatt.
p.   cm.
Includes bibliographical references and index.
ISBN 0-8342-0550-5
1. Neuromuscular diseases—Diagnosis. 2. Diagnosis, Differential.
I. Title.
[DNLM: 1. Musculoskeletal Diseases—diagnosis—handbooks.
2. Chiropractic—methods—handbooks. 3. Diagnosis, Differential—
handbooks. WE 39 W975d 1994]
RC925.7.W93   1994
616.7'075—dc20
DNLM/DLC
for Library of Congress
94-1815
CIP

The authors have made every effort to ensure the accuracy of the information herein, particularly with regard to technique and procedure.
However, appropriate information sources should be consulted, especially for new or unfamiliar procedures. It is the responsibility of every
practitioner to evaluate the appropriateness of a particular opinion in
the context of actual clinical situations and with due consideration to
new developments. Authors, editors, and the publisher cannot be held
responsible for any typographical or other errors found in this book.

Editorial Resources: Amy R. Martin

Library of Congress Catalog Card Number: 94-1815
ISBN: 0-8342-0550-5

Printed in the United States of America

1   2   3   4   5

To my beloved wife Cheryl
Never has there been a more perfect companion

Table of Contents

Preface

Differential diagnosis is, in my opinion, the one true "art" in health care. One of the most difficult tasks facing any physician is the collation of seemingly endless large groups of apparently unrelated facts related to patient presentation into a logical list of probable diagnoses.

During my tenure as an educator and administrator involved in the training of chiropractic physicians, it has become apparent that a quick reference text aimed at the differential diagnosis of common neuromusculoskeletal disorders is needed. There are many texts on differential diagnosis of neurologic, muscular, and skeletal disorders, and those authors are to be commended. They are not designed with the combination of these entities in one manuscript for use by the physician presented with these conditions on a daily basis.

This handbook is designed to provide the reader with rapid access to the differential diagnosis of the more commonly seen neuromusculoskeletal disorders in general clinical practice. It is certainly not all-inclusive in scope.

Part I provides lists of differential diagnoses for neurologic signs and symptoms and for radiographic signs. Part II supplies the reader with lists that are a helpful adjunct to Part I. In Part III, specific disease presentations are outlined in list format. It is understood that some readers will find the lists in-complete. The differential diagnosis lists have been modified to make quick reference more easily accomplished by listing only those diseases that are seen not uncommonly in a general fam-ily practice. Where appropriate, the lists are organized by etiol-ogy. But when this is not possible, other categorization schemes have been used.

A basic knowledge of neuromusculoskeletal diagnosis and the art of differential diagnosis is assumed. The reader is pro-vided with a bibliography that will further elucidate the sub-jects covered. Illustrations have been provided as an adjunct to differential diagnosis.

The reader is invited to submit other lists or modifications to the presented lists that you believe are pertinent to the subject matter.

I hope you will use this text until the cover is worn and tat-tered and then use it some more. I hope it is highlighted in five different colors and written in in three different colored inks. I hope it becomes your own personal "teratoma" that never leaves your side.

How To Use This Book

This text is organized into three sections: differential diagnosis, helpful lists, and selected disorders. It is made specifically as a quick reference for the clinician confronted with signs, symptoms, and radiographic findings that present a diagnostic challenge. It is best utilized by locating each of the signs, symptoms, and radiographic findings in the Table of Contents and text and cross-referencing the differential diagnosis lists to formulate an appropriate final differential diagnosis. Each of the more common and life-threatening disorders may then be located in the section on disorders where more in-depth information is found.

Normally, the lists of disorders are organized by etiology (e.g., vascular, trauma) and, where appropriate, the most common cause of a sign or symptom is noted by the abbreviation m.c. It should be remembered that there are many instances where the most common cause of a finding will eventually be the final diagnosis, but more life-threatening causes must first be ruled out.

Illustrations are provided as an adjunct where they are often helpful in formulating a diagnosis.

Acknowledgments

This is my second textbook, and I can truthfully say that, other than layout, this book was no easier than the first. The accomplishment of this manuscript did not happen without much assistance and support.

I am forever indebted to all those who helped, but I must thank a few unique individuals: Martha Sasser, "Thanks for asking again"; Dr. T. Sammi Lowe, "Thanks for being an inspiration and a role model"; Dr. Cheri' Lane, "You are truly outstanding"; and to my wife, "Moofie, thanks for putting up with me again. You're the greatest and I love you!" To Dr. Joseph Howe, I give my gratitude and love for being my mentor. I also thank Dr. Kiki Kilpatrick for her "awesome" artwork. Amy Martin, thank you so much for your guidance and advice, but most of all thank you for your enthusiasm. You are one of a kind. The summer of 1992 was indeed an experience!

Part I

Differential Diagnosis

Chapter 1

Cranial Nerve Disorders

DIFFERENTIAL DIAGNOSIS BASED ON CLINICAL FINDINGS

1.1 Cranial Nerve I (Olfactory) Lesions

Signs/Symptoms

Anosmia

Clinical Notes

Unilateral anosmia; think structural/obstructing lesion

Differential Diagnosis

- Vascular
    Infarction (anterior cerebral artery distribution)
    Arteriovenous malformation (frontal lobe)
- Tumors
    Frontal lobe masses
    Sinus/nasal mass
- Idiopathic
    Smoking
    Normal aging process

- Metabolic
  Diabetes mellitus
  Hypothyroidism
- Trauma (cribriform plate m.c.)
- Infection
  Chronic rhinitis
  Chronic sinusitis
- Miscellaneous
  Associated with aging

1.2 Cranial Nerve II (Optic) Lesions

Signs/Symptoms

Blindness
Visual field defects (Figures 1-1 and 1-2)
Papilledema

Clinical Notes

Disc swelling with abnormal vision; anterior lesions
Normal disc with abnormal vision; posterior (retrobulbar)
  lesions
Disc swelling with normal vision; think papilledema
Must be distinguished from intraorbital and intrinsic eye
  disease
Rapid onset; think aneurysm
Slow onset; think metabolic disease

Differential Diagnosis

- Tumors
  Orbital

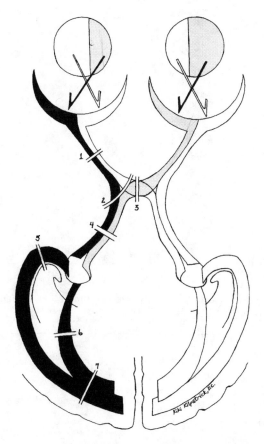

Note: Numbered lesions correspond to visual field defects in Figure 1-2.

Figure 1-1 Central Nervous System Vision Pathways with Typical Lesions.
Source: Copyright © 1993 by Kiki Kilpatrick, D.C.

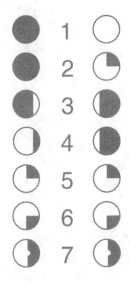

Figure 1-2 Visual Field Defects that Correspond to Lesions in Figure 1-1.
Source: Copyright © 1993 by Kiki Kilpatrick, D.C.

  Sellar/parasellar
  Chiasmal
  Optic nerve/sheath
- Vascular
  Infarction
- Metabolic
  Diabetes mellitus
  Hyperthyroidism

- Inflammation
  Optic neuritis
- Demyelination
  Multiple sclerosis
- Trauma

1.3 Cranial Nerve III (Oculomotor) Palsy

Signs/Symptoms

Weakness of superior/inferior/medial rectus and/or
  superior oblique muscles
Mydriasis
Ptosis

Clinical Notes

Bilateral palsies; think systemic disease (e.g.,
  hyperthyroidism, myasthenia gravis)
+/- Exophthalmos

Differential Diagnosis

- Vascular
  Infarction
  Aneurysm (m.c., posterior cerebral artery, internal
    carotid artery)
  Cavernous sinus thrombosis
  Migraine headache
- Tumor
  Pituitary adenoma
  Meningioma
  Intraorbital

- Inflammation
    Meningitis
    Guillain-Barré syndrome
    Inflammatory vasculopathy
- Trauma
    Orbital fractures

1.4 Cranial Nerve IV (Trochlear) Palsy

Signs/Symptoms

Superior and nasal deviation of the affected eye
Isolated trochlear palsy is rare

Clinical Notes

May mimic strabismus

Differential Diagnosis

- Vascular
    Infarction
    Hemorrhage
    Aneurysm
    Cavernous sinus thrombosis
- Tumor
    Meningioma
    Pinealoma
- Inflammation
    Meningitis
    Ethmoiditis
    Mastoiditis

- Trauma
    Brainstem
    Eye

1.5 Cranial Nerve V (Trigeminal) Lesions

Signs/Symptoms

Brief paroxysms of severe trigeminal distribution pain

Clinical Notes

Most common type of facial neuralgia
Sensory/motor examination normal in idiopathic form
Sensory/motor abnormalities in symptomatic form
90% occur after age 40 years

Differential Diagnosis

- Vascular (posterior fossa)
    Aneurysm
    Arteriovenous malformation
- Tumor (posterior fossa)
    Acoustic neuroma
    Meningioma
    Trigeminal neuroma
- Metabolic
    Diabetes mellitus
- Inflammation
    Progressive systemic sclerosis
    Systemic lupus erythematosus
    Sjögren's syndrome
    Herpes

- Demyelination
  Multiple sclerosis
- Idiopathic
  Tic douloureux
- Trauma
  Facial trauma

1.6 Cranial Nerve VI (Abducens) Palsy

Signs/Symptoms

Internal strabismus
Diplopia

Clinical Notes

Most common type of external ocular palsy

Differential Diagnosis

- Vascular
  Aneurysm (m.c., anterior inferior cerebellar artery,
    basilar artery)
  Subarachnoid hemorrhage
  Infarction
  Cavernous sinus thrombosis
  Migraine headache
- Tumor
  Pontine glioma
  Cerebellar
  Acoustic neuroma
  Chordoma

  Meningioma
  Pituitary adenoma
- Inflammation
  Meningitis
  Mastoiditis
  Petrositis
- Miscellaneous
  After lumbar puncture (e.g., myelogram)
- Demyelination
  Multiple sclerosis

1.7 Cranial Nerve VII (Facial) Palsy

Signs/Symptoms

 Weakness of muscles of facial expression

Clinical Notes

 Inability to close eyes completely; think peripheral lesion

Differential Diagnosis

- Idiopathic (m.c.)
  Bell's palsy (m.c. peripheral nerve palsy)
- Trauma
  Facial fracture
  Skull fracture
  Surgery
- Tumor
  Schwannoma
  Neurofibroma
  Parotid gland

- Infection
    Petrositis
    Mastoiditis
    Otitis media
    Facial neuritis

1.8 Cranial Nerve VIII (Vestibulocochlear) Lesions

Signs/Symptoms

Hearing loss
Tinnitus
Vertigo

Differential Diagnosis

- Hearing loss
    Tumors (e.g., acoustic neuroma)
    Meningitis
    Drugs (e.g., aspirin, aminoglycosides, furosemide)
    Multiple sclerosis
    Infection (e.g., virus)
    Paget's disease
- Tinnitus
    Presbycusis
    Trauma
    Tumors (e.g., acoustic neuroma)
- Vertigo
    Vestibular neuritis
    Labyrinthitis
    Drugs (similar to hearing loss above)
    Tumors

Multiple sclerosis
Infection (e.g., virus)
- Trauma

1.9 Cranial Nerves IX, X, and XI (Glossopharyngeal, Vagus, Spinal Accessory) Lesions

Signs/Symptoms

Dysphagia (liquids more than solids)
Dysarthria
Hoarseness
Uvular deviation
Weakness of sternocleidomastoid or trapezius muscles

Clinical Notes

Seen also with bulbar palsy
Lesions are usually of the brainstem

Differential Diagnosis

- Tumor
  Glioma
  Metastasis
  Syringobulbia
- Vascular
  Infarction
  Hemorrhage
  Vertebral artery aneurysm
- Inflammation
  Meningitis
  Encephalitis

- Demyelination
    Multiple sclerosis

1.10 Cranial Nerve XII (Hypoglossal) Lesions

Signs/Symptoms

Tongue deviation/weakness

Clinical Notes

Tongue deviates to involved side

Differential Diagnosis

- Tumor
    Brainstem glioma
    Metastasis
    Osseous tumors of the skull base (e.g., chordoma)
    Syringobulbia
- Vascular
    Infarction
    Hemorrhage
    Aneurysm
- Congenital
    Arnold-Chiari malformation
    Basilar invagination
- Inflammation
    Meningitis
    Nasopharyngitis
- Demyelination
    Multiple sclerosis

1.11 Cranial Nerve Functions (Figure 1-3)

Nerve	Functions
I (Olfactory)	Smell
II (Optic)	Visual acuity
III (Oculomotor)	Superior, medial, and inferior eye motions
	Pupillary constriction
IV (Trochlear)	Inferolateral eye motion (superior oblique muscle)
V (Trigeminal)	Facial sensation (3 branches: V1, V2, V3)
	Muscles of mastication (motor)
VI (Abducens)	Lateral eye motion (lateral rectus)
VII (Facial)	Muscles of facial expression (motor)
	Taste on anterior two-thirds of tongue
	Salivation and tearing
	Sensation of inner ear
	Stapedius muscle innervation
VIII (Vestibulocochlear)	Hearing
	Vestibular function
IX (Glossopharyngeal)	Sensation on posterior tongue/pharynx
	Taste on posterior one-third of tongue
	Salivation
	Stylopharyngeus muscle (motor)
X (Vagus)	Visceral parasympathetic innervation
	Pharyngeal/laryngeal muscles (motor)
XI (Spinal Accessory)	Trapezius/sternocleidomastoid muscles (motor)
XII (Hypoglossal)	Muscles of tongue (motor)

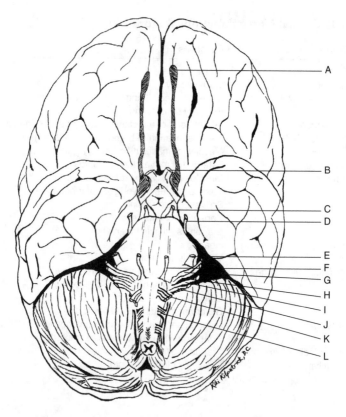

A
B
C
D
E
F
G
H
I
J
K
L

Note: (A) olfactory; (B) optic; (C) oculomotor; (D) trochlear; (E) trigeminal; (F) abducens; (G) facial; (H) vestibulocochlear; (I) glossopharyngeal; (J) vagus; (K) hypoglossal; (L) spinal accessory.

Figure 1-3 Base of the Brain with Cranial Nerves. *Source:* Copyright © 1993 by Kiki Kilpatrick, D.C.

Chapter 2

Neuromuscular Disorders

DIFFERENTIAL DIAGNOSIS BASED ON CLINICAL FINDINGS

2.1 Agnosia

Failure to recognize a stimulus in a person with intact primary sensation

Clinical Notes

Astereognosis (see also 2.6)—inability to recognize object placed in the hands

Agraphesthesia—inability to identify number drawn on the skin

Usually contralateral to hemispheric lesion

Symptoms of sensory loss are isolated to the area of disturbed cerebral function (e.g., visual, tactile)

Differential Diagnosis

- Vascular
    Cerebrovascular accident (m.c.)
    Hemorrhage
- Tumor
    Cerebral

2.2 Amaurosis Fugax

Transient monocular blindness from retinal ischemia

Clinical Notes

Sudden onset and short duration (< 30 minutes)
Black or gray color

Differential Diagnosis

- Vascular
    Embolization of ophthalmic artery (m.c.) or internal
        carotid artery
    Stenosis of ophthalmic artery
    Hypertensive crisis
    Giant cell arteritis
- Ocular disease
    Glaucoma
    Optic nerve edema (papilledema)
- Demyelination
    Multiple sclerosis
- Miscellaneous
    Migraine

2.3 Amnesia

Loss of memory

Differential Diagnosis

- Trauma
    Head trauma (m.c.)

- Vascular
    Ischemia (especially posterior cerebral artery)
    Cerebrovascular accident
- Transient global amnesia
- Dementias
- Tumors (rare)
    Cerebral
- Epilepsy

2.4 Anisocoria

Difference of more than 1 mm in pupillary size from right
   to left

Differential Diagnosis

- Vascular
    Cerebrovascular accident
    Ischemia
    Migraine headache
- Congenital
    Anomaly (without clinical significance)
- Tumor
    Pancoasts tumor with Horner's syndrome
    Cranial nerve III tumor
    Brain tumor with cranial nerve III compression
- Inflammation
    Ciliary ganglionitis
    Pupillatonia (Adie's pupil)
- Trauma
    Cervical spine (Claude Bernard syndrome)

2.5 Aphasia

Inability to communicate, especially with speech

Clinical Notes

Expressive form—good comprehension, poor fluency
Receptive form—poor comprehension, good fluency
Usually from left hemispheric lesion (with right-handed-
ness)

Differential Diagnosis

- Vascular
    Cerebrovascular accident (m.c.)
    Arteriovenous malformation
- Tumor
    Cerebral

2.6 Astereognosis

Inability to recognize touched objects

Clinical Notes

Lesions of contralateral cerebral hemisphere, especially
superior parietal lobe and thalamoparietal tracts

Differential Diagnosis

- Vascular
    Cerebrovascular accident (m.c.)
- Tumor
    Cerebral

2.7 Ataxia

Lack of muscular coordination and precision motor tasks

Clinical Notes

Usually associated with cerebellar disease
Also seen with posterior column disease, neuropathies
Diffuse abnormal proprioception may mimic ataxia
Dysdiadochokinesia and dysmetria are common associations

Differential Diagnosis

- Vascular
    Cerebrovascular accident
    Migraine
    Hemorrhage
    Arteriovenous malformation
- Tumor
    Posterior fossa neoplasms
    Arachnoid cyst
    Dandy-Walker cyst
- Demyelination
    Multiple sclerosis
- Infection
    Viral
- Degenerative
    Friedreich's ataxia
    Ataxia-telangiectasia
- Metabolic
    Alcoholism/Wernicke-Korsakoff syndrome

Heavy metal poisoning (mercury)
Hepatic encephalopathy
Hypothyroidism

2.8 Behavioral Abnormalities

Change in normal behavior

Differential Diagnosis

- Tumor
    Cerebral
- Epilepsy
- Alcoholism
- Vascular
    Cerebrovascular accident
    Ischemia
- Dementias
- Senescence

2.9 Blackouts

See Syncope, Drop attacks

2.10 Choreoathetosis

Clinical Notes

Chorea—involuntary rapid jerky movements
Athetosis—involuntary slow writhing movements
Disappears during sleep; aggravated by stress

Differential Diagnosis

- Vascular
    Cerebrovascular accident
    Migraine
    Arteriovenous malformation
    Hemorrhage
- Tumor
    Cerebral
- Demyelination
    Multiple sclerosis
- Metabolic
    Diabetes mellitus
    Hyperthyroidism
    Hypoglycemia
    Pregnancy (chorea gravidarum)
    Electrolyte imbalance
    Alcoholism
    Drugs (e.g., neuroleptics, oral contraceptive agent,
      steroids)
    Vitamin B deficiency
    Hepatic/renal diseases
- Infection
    Syndenham's chorea
    Lyme disease
    Creutzfeldt-Jakob disease
- Degenerative
    Huntington's disease
    Senile chorea
    Ataxia-telangiectasia

- Congenital
    Benign hereditary chorea
    Tuberous sclerosis
    Lesch-Nyhan syndrome
    Niemann-Pick disease
- Trauma
    Concussion
    Hematoma (epidural/subdural)

2.11 Claudication

Achy pain in the extremities with sustained motion

Clinical Notes

Flexion of the spine may relieve neurogenic form but not
    vascular form
Both forms relieved by rest

Differential Diagnosis

- Vascular (lower extremity only)
    Occlusion of aorta and/or tributaries
    Abdominal aortic aneurysm
- Neurogenic (upper and lower extremities)
    Spinal canal stenosis

2.12 Clonus

Irregular, brief, involuntary muscle contractions

Clinical Notes

May be precipitated by sensory stimuli or passive move-
    ment

Differential Diagnosis

- Physiologic
    Anxiety
    Sleep jerks
    Exercise
- Myelopathy
    Spinal canal stenosis
    Cauda equina syndrome
    Conus medullaris syndrome
- Idiopathic
    Hereditary benign
    Nocturnal myoclonus
- Vascular
    After cerebrovascular accident
- Tumor
    Cerebral
    Spinal cord
- Inflammatory
    Encephalitis
- Neurodegenerative
    Parkinson's disease
    Alzheimer's disease
- Head trauma
- Psychologic
- Metabolic
    Hypo/hyperglycemia
    Drug ingestion
    Heavy metal poisoning

2.13 Cogwheel Phenomenon

Jerky and resisted joint range of motion

Clinical Notes

Especially common at the wrist

Differential Diagnosis

- Extrapyramidal syndromes
    Parkinson's disease
    Chorea
    Athetosis
    Dystonias (e.g., spastic torticollis)
    Wilson's disease (hepatolenticular degeneration)

2.14 Convulsions

See Seizures

2.15 Deafness

Sensorineural hearing loss

Clinical Notes

Exclude conduction loss first
Magnetic resonance imaging is an excellent diagnostic tool
    for unilateral deafness

Differential Diagnosis

- Tumor
    Acoustic neuroma

      Glomus jugulare tumor
      Arachnoid cyst
- Neuroectodermal syndromes (Phakomatoses)
      Neurofibromatosis
- Infection
      Mumps
      Herpes zoster
      Meningitis
- Trauma
- Demyelination
      Multiple sclerosis
- Drugs
      Aspirin
      Aminoglycosides
      Diuretics
- Miscellaneous
      Meniere's disease

2.16 Dementia

Impaired learning, memory, cognition with disorientation

Differential Diagnosis

- Degenerative
      Alzheimer's disease (m.c.)
- Vascular
      Multiple infarctions
      Chronic subdural hematoma
- Tumor
      Cerebral
- Hydrocephalus

- Demyelination
    Multiple sclerosis
    Leukodystrophies
- Metabolic
    Hypothyroidism
    Alcoholism/Wernicke-Korsakoff syndrome
    Vitamin B-12 deficiency
    Pellagra (Nicotinic acid deficiency)
    Hypercalcemia
    Drug ingestion
    Heavy metal poisoning (lead)
- Infection
    Human immunodeficiency virus
    Meningitis (chronic)
- Trauma
- Psychogenic
- Epilepsy

2.17 Diplopia

Double vision

Differential Diagnosis

- Ophthalmoplegia
- Vascular
    Intracranial aneurysm
    Arteriovenous malformation
- Tumor
    Cerebral

2.18 Dizziness

See Syncope, Dysequilibrium, Light-headedness, Vertigo

2.19 Drop Attacks (see also **Syncope, Light-headedness**)

Unconsciousness without permanent neurologic deficit

Clinical Notes

Short duration (usually only a few minutes)

Differential Diagnosis

- Vascular
    Vertebrobasilar artery insufficiency (m.c.)
- Cardiac disease
    Tachycardias
    Sick sinus syndrome
- Cataplexy (paroxysmal loss of muscle tone)

2.20 Dysequilibrium

Loss of balance without subjective movement sensations of
    the head

Differential Diagnosis

- Cerebellar disease
- Posterior column disease
- Muscle weakness

2.21 Dysmetria

Inappropriate amplitude and tempo of intentional movements

Clinical Notes

Excessive splaying of fingers when grasping a small object

Differential Diagnosis

- Cerebellar disease

2.22 Dysphagia

Difficulty in swallowing

Clinical Notes

Liquids worse than solids suggests neurologic disease
Solids worse than liquids suggests obstructive disease of
esophagus
Neurologic diseases only listed below

Differential Diagnosis

- Tumor
    Brainstem neoplasms
    Compressive cerebral neoplasms
- Dystrophies
    Myotonic dystrophy
    Oculopharyngeal dystrophy

- Demyelination
    Multiple sclerosis
- Syringobulbia

2.23 Epilepsy

See Seizures

2.24 Fasciculations

Contractions of large groups of muscle fibers

Clinical Notes

Can be seen as a twitch under the skin

Differential Diagnosis

- Endocrine/metabolic
    Hypokalemia
    Hypocalcemia
    Hyperthyroidism
    Uremia
    Heavy metal poisoning
- Neurologic
    Amyotrophic lateral sclerosis
    Syringomyelia
    Poliomyelitis
    Spinal cord infarction
    Radiculopathy
- Arthritides
    Spinal canal stenosis from degenerative joint disease

- Trauma
    Spinal cord
- Tumor
    Spinal cord
- Drugs
    Cholinergics

2.25 Footdrop

Differential Diagnosis

- Palsies
    Common peroneal nerve palsy
    Sciatic nerve palsy
- Nerve root lesions
    L4
    L5
- Peripheral neuropathy
    Diabetes mellitus
- Central nervous system disease
    Cerebrovascular accident
- Myopathy

2.26 Headache

Clinical Notes

Classification is by etiology

Differential Diagnosis

- Muscle tension (m.c.)
- Vascular
    Migraine (atypical, common, classic)
    Premenstrual
    Cluster (typical, chronic)
    Paroxysmal hemicrania
    Hypertension
    Hemorrhage
    Hematoma
    Cerebrovascular accident
    Aneurysm
    Arteriovenous malformation
- Arthritides
    Cervical spine degenerative joint disease
- Tumor
    Brain
    Upper cervical spinal cord
- Inflammation
    Meningitis
    Cerebral abscess
    Encephalitis
    Vasculitis
- Metabolic
    Fever
    Hypoglycemia
    Drug ingestion
- Miscellaneous
    Cervical subluxation (especially C2/3)

      Cervical degenerative joint disease
      Pseudotumor cerebri
      Temporomandibular joint disease
      Dental disease
      Cough headache
      Exercise
      Postcoital headache
      Ocular disease
      Nasal/sinus disease
      Postmyelogram
- Psychogenic

2.27 Hearing Loss

See Deafness

2.28 Horner's Syndrome

Clinical Notes

Unilateral ptosis, meiosis, anhydrosis

Differential Diagnosis

- Tumor
      Pancoast's tumor
      Thyroid
      Pharyngeal
      Spinal cord
      Mediastinal
- Trauma

- Cluster headache
- Postsurgical
- Vascular
- Cervical disc herniation

2.29 Hydrocephalus

Hindrance of normal cerebrospinal fluid circulation

Clinical Notes

Obstructive (no communication between ventricles and subarachnoid space)
Communicating (normal communication)

Differential Diagnosis (Obstructive)

- Tumor
    Third ventricle
    Fourth ventricle
    Posterior fossa
- Congenital
    Arnold-Chiari malformation
    Obstruction of aqueduct of Sylvius or foramina
    Meningiomyelocele

Differential Diagnosis (Communicating)

- Vascular
    Hemorrhage
    Hematoma
- Infection
    Meningitis

- Miscellaneous
    Cerebral atrophy (pseudohydrocephalus)
    Venous sinus thrombosis

2.30 Hyperreflexia

Increased deep tendon reflexes

Clinical Notes

Seen mainly with upper motor neuron lesions
Result of loss of corticospinal inhibition

Differential Diagnosis

- Vascular
    Cerebrovascular accident
    Hemorrhage
    Hematoma
    Arteriovenous malformation
- Tumor
    Cerebral
    Brainstem
    Spinal cord
- Miscellaneous
    Spinal canal stenosis
- Trauma

2.31 Hyporeflexia

Decreased deep tendon reflexes

Clinical Notes

Early sign in upper motor neuron lesions
Seen throughout in lower motor neuron lesions

Differential Diagnosis

- Neuropathy
    Radiculopathy (typically unilateral)
    Polyneuropathy (typically bilateral)
    Peripheral nerve entrapment
- Tumor
    Spinal cord (early)
- Vascular
    Cerebrovascular accident
- Muscular disease
    Polymyositis
- Inflammation
    Guillain-Barré syndrome

2.32 Impotence

Inability to obtain or maintain an erection

Clinical Notes

Categorized in functional and organic causes

Differential Diagnosis

- Metabolic
    Diabetes mellitus
    Pituitary disease

- Vascular
    Atherosclerosis
    Arteritis
    Priapism
    Thromboembolic disease
- Spinal cord disease
    Tumor
    Trauma
    Spinal canal stenosis
- Demyelination
    Multiple sclerosis
- Degenerative
    Parkinson's disease
- Postsurgical
    Bladder
    Prostate
- Inflammation
    Urinary tract infection
- Structural abnormalities
    Obesity
    Peyronie's disease
- Drugs
    Antihypertensives
- Psychogenic

2.33 Incontinence

Loss of bowel or bladder control

Differential Diagnosis

- Tumor
    Spinal cord
    Cerebral
- Trauma
    Spinal cord
    Brain
- Spinal canal stenosis
- Postsurgical
- Senescence
- Metabolic
    Diabetes mellitus
- Miscellaneous
    Amyotrophic lateral sclerosis

2.34 Light-headedness

Differential Diagnosis

- Miscellaneous
    Hyperventilation
    Multiple sensory deficits (e.g., visual and vestibular
        dysfunction)
    Psychogenic
    Anemia
    Carotid sinus hypersensitivity
- Drugs
    Antiarrythmics
    Anticonvulsants
    Antidepressants

> Antihistamines
> Antihypertensives
> Alcohol
> Tobacco

- Metabolic
  > Hypoglycemia
  > Addison's disease
- Trauma
  > Head
  > Cervical spine
- Vascular
  > Vertebrobasilar artery insufficiency

2.35 Meiosis

Bilateral pupillary constriction

Differential Diagnosis

- Senescence
- Drugs
- Pontine lesions
- Argyll Robertson pupils
- Normal variant

2.36 Memory Loss

See Amnesia

2.37 Multiple Cranial Nerve Palsies

Differential Diagnosis

- Tumor
    Nasopharyngeal carcinoma
    Brainstem tumors
- Infection
    Meningitis
- Metabolic/endocrine
    Diabetes mellitus
- Miscellaneous
    Guillain-Barré syndrome
    Paget's disease
    Arnold-Chiari malformation
- Trauma

2.38 Muscle Cramps

Sudden, involuntary, painful muscle contraction

Differential Diagnosis

- Trauma
    Overuse
    Exercise
    "Charley horse"
    Peripheral nerve injury
- Neuropathy
    Nerve root compression
    Motor neuropathy
    Peripheral nerve entrapment

- Metabolic
    Uremia
    Hypoglycemia
    Hypocalcemia
    Hyponatremia
    Hypo/hyperkalemia
    Hypomagnesemia
    Respiratory alkalosis
- Drugs
    Calcium channel blockers (e.g., nifedipine)
    Alcohol
    Beta-agonists (e.g., terbutaline)
- Miscellaneous
    Nocturnal leg cramps
    Heat cramps
    Old poliomyelitis

2.39 Muscle Weakness (Chronic Generalized)

Differential Diagnosis

- Endocrine/metabolic
    Hypo/hyperthyroidism
    Acromegaly
    Vitamin D deficiency
    Electrolyte imbalance
    Hyperparathyroidism
- Neurologic
    Amyotrophic lateral sclerosis
    Guillain-Barré syndrome
    Myasthenia gravis

- Myopathy
  Polymyositis
  Dermatomyositis
- Infection
  Toxoplasmosis
  Cysticercosis
  Trichinosis
- Drugs/toxins
  Beta-blockers (e.g., propranolol)
  Lithium
  Corticosteroids
  Alcohol
- Miscellaneous
  Amyloidosis
  Sarcoidosis

2.40 Myalgia

Muscular pain and discomfort

Differential Diagnosis

- Trauma
  Direct
  Overuse (m.c.)
- Vascular
  Intermittent claudication
- Inflammation/infection
  Viral
  Bacterial
  Connective tissue disorders (e.g., rheumatoid arthritis,
      scleroderma)

Fibromyalgia syndrome
Thrombophlebitis

- Metabolic/endocrine
  Electrolyte imbalance (e.g., calcium, potassium,
      sodium, magnesium)
  Hypothyroidism
  Enzyme defects (e.g., myophosphorylase deficiency
      [McArdle's disease])
  Pregnancy

- Drugs
  Alcohol
  Amphetamines
  Cytotoxic drugs (e.g., vincristine)
  Cimetidine
  Diuretics
  Tetanus

- Neurologic
  Primary myopathy (e.g., myotonia congenita)
  Neuropathy (e.g., neuritis)
  Amyotrophic lateral sclerosis
  Parkinson's disease
  Multiple sclerosis
  "Stiff man" syndrome
  Reflex spasm from nerve irritation

2.41 Mydriasis

Bilateral pupillary dilatation

Differential Diagnosis

- Drugs
- Psychogenic (e.g., pain)
- Hyperthyroidism
- Seizures
- Blindness
- Normal variant

2.42 Myelopathy

Lesion affecting the spinal cord causing upper motor
  neuron lesion

Differential Diagnosis

- Congenital
    Spinal dysraphism
    Basilar invagination
    Spinal canal stenosis
- Trauma
    Syringomyelia
    Fracture/dislocation
    Subluxation with cord compression
    Disc protrusion/extrusion
    Cord compression/contusion
- Tumor
    Extramedullary (e.g., meningioma)
    Intramedullary (e.g., ependymoma)
- Infection
    Abscess

    Fungal
    Meningitis
- Arthritides
    Degenerative joint disease with spinal canal stenosis
    Inflammatory arthropathy
    Ossification of the posterior longitudinal ligament
- Vascular
    Infarction
    Hemorrhage
    Arteriovenous malformation
- Metabolic
    Pernicious anemia
    Nicotinic acid deficiency
    Chronic liver disease

2.43 Neck Stiffness

Differential Diagnosis

- Arthritides
    Degenerative joint disease
    Diffuse idiopathic skeletal hyperostosis
    Ossification of the posterior longitudinal ligament
    Inflammatory arthritides
- Neuropathy
    Nerve root compression
    Peripheral neuropathy
    Reflex muscle spasm from nerve irritation
- Miscellaneous
    Cervical spine subluxation

- Trauma
    Sprain/strain
- Infection
    Meningitis
    Spinal epidural abscess
- Vascular
    Hemorrhage

2.44 Neuropathy

Focal peripheral neuronal lesions

Differential Diagnosis

- Trauma
- Arthritides
    Degenerative joint disease
    Inflammatory arthropathy
- Infection
    Syphilis
    Tuberculosis
    Herpes zoster
- Vascular
    Arteritis
    Sickle cell anemia
    Polycythemia
    Hemophilia
    Thromboembolic disease (e.g., thromboangiitis
        obliterans)
- Tumor
    Nerve fiber/sheath (e.g., schwannoma)

Lymphoma
Leukemia
Metastasis
- Metabolic
  Diabetes mellitus
  Heavy metal poisoning

2.45 Nystagmus

Rapid alternating involuntary movements of the eye(s)

Clinical Notes

Defined by fast component of alternating movement
May be horizontal, vertical, or rotary

Differential Diagnosis

- Congenital
  Arnold-Chiari malformation
  Congenital nystagmus
  Basilar invagination
- Tumor
  Cerebellum
  Pons
  Brainstem
- Demyelination
  Multiple sclerosis
- Ocular disease
  Amblyopia
  Strabismus
- Drugs
- Myasthenia gravis

2.46 Orthostatic Hypotension (see also **Syncope**)

Greater than 10 mm Hg decrease in blood pressure from recumbent to upright posture

Clinical Notes

Light-headedness
Fainting
Precipitated by rapid changes in position

Differential Diagnosis

- Drugs/poisons
    Alcohol
    Diuretics
    Calcium channel blockers
    Nitrates
    Narcotic analgesics
    Sedatives
    Tricyclic antidepressants
    Phenobarbital
- Neurologic
    Cerebrovascular accident
    Tumor
    Parkinson's disease
    Diabetic neuropathy
    Guillain-Barré syndrome
- Cardiac
    Congestive heart failure
    Mitral valve prolapse
- Endocrine
    Hypoadrenalism

Diabetes insipidus
Pheochromocytoma
Hypoaldosteronism
- Miscellaneous
Idiopathic
Dehydration
Severe anemia
Prolonged bedrest

2.47 Palsy

See Chapters 1 and 4 for specific palsies

2.48 Papilledema

Swelling of the optic disc

Differential Diagnosis

- Tumor (m.c.)
Intracranial
Optic nerve
- Vascular
Venous thrombosis
Subarachnoid hemorrhage
- Trauma
Subdural hematoma
- Infection
Brain abscess
Meningitis
Encephalitis

- Outflow obstruction
    Craniocervical anomalies
    Aqueduct stenosis
- Miscellaneous
    Pseudotumor cerebri

2.49 Paralysis

Loss of the power of movement

Clinical Notes

Spastic—paralysis with muscle hypertonicity
Flaccid—paralysis with no muscle tone

Differential Diagnosis

- Spastic
    Upper motor neuron lesions
- Flaccid
    Lower motor neuron lesions

2.50 Polyneuropathy

Disturbance of multiple peripheral nerves

Differential Diagnosis

- Metabolic/nutritional
    Diabetes mellitus (m.c.)
    Vitamin B-12 deficiency
    Uremia
    Cirrhosis of the liver
    Malabsorption syndromes

- Toxins
    Alcohol
    Lead
    Drugs (e.g., isoniazid)
- Congenital
    Charcot-Marie-Tooth disease
    Porphyria
    Primary amyloidosis
- Tumor
    Metastasis
- Infection
    Parotitis
    Mononucleosis
    Botulism
    Human immunodeficiency virus
    Herpes zoster

2.51 Ptosis

Drooping of the upper eyelid (Figure 2-1)

Clinical Notes

True ptosis—disease of levator palpebrae muscle or innervation of the muscle
Pseudoptosis—causes other than true ptosis

Differential Diagnosis

- Congenital
    Idiopathic
    Orbital tumor

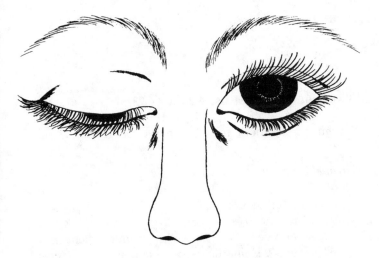

Figure 2-1 Ptosis of the Right Upper Eyelid. *Source:* Copyright © 1993 by Kiki Kilpatrick, D.C.

- Myopathy
    Myasthenia gravis
    Polymyositis
    Topical steroid eye drops
- Cranial nerve III lesions
- Pseudoptosis
    Horner's syndrome
    Allergies
    Blepharitis
    Conjunctivitis
    Chronic Bell's palsy

2.52 Pupil Inequality

See Anisocoria

2.53 Radiculopathy (see also **4.22** and **4.23**)

Extremity dysesthesia from true nerve root lesion

Differential Diagnosis

- Intervertebral disc disease
    Disc protrusion/extrusion
    Degenerative joint disease with foraminal stenosis
    Degenerative joint disease with lateral recess stenosis
- Tumors
    Neurofibroma
    Neuroma of the cauda equina
    Metastasis
- Trauma
- Vascular
    Epidural hematoma
- Congenital
    Spinal canal stenosis
- Miscellaneous
    Herpes zoster

2.54 Seizures

Categorized by age

Differential Diagnosis

- Infants
    Fever
    Trauma
    Infection
    Idiopathic
- Childhood
    Trauma
    Infection
    Arteriovenous malformation
- Adolescence
    Idiopathic
    Trauma
    Drug withdrawal
    Brain tumor
    Arteriovenous malformation
- Adult
    Brain tumor
    Cerebrovascular disease
    Alcoholism
    Hypoglycemia
    Trauma
    Infection of the central nervous system
    Drug-induced

2.55 Syncope

Temporary loss of consciousness and postural tone; fainting

Differential Diagnosis

- Hypotension
    Vasovagal response
    Orthostatic hypotension
    Carotid sinus syndrome
    Micturition syncope
    Defecation syncope
    Cough syncope
    Swallow syncope
    Hypovolemia
    Medications (e.g., nitrates)
- Cardiac disease
    Valvular disease (e.g., aortic stenosis)
    Arrhythmias (e.g., atrial fibrillation, sick sinus syndrome)
    Myocardial infarction
- Cerebral disease
    Ischemia
    Seizures
- Psychiatric
    Hysterical
    Hyperventilation
- Metabolic
- Miscellaneous
    Subclavian steal syndrome
    Pulmonary embolism

2.56 Tinnitus

Sensation of ringing in the ear(s)

Clinical Notes

Subjective—heard only by patients
Objective—may be heard by examiner

Differential Diagnosis

- Miscellaneous
    Physiologic
    Presbycusis
    Meniere's disease
    Fever
    Tobacco
    Ethanol
    Increased intracranial pressure
    Ototoxic drugs
    Excess cerumen
    Temporomandibular joint disorders
    Otosclerosis
- Vascular
    Hypertension
    Intracranial aneurysm
    Venous sinus thrombosis
    Aortic valvular disease
    Arteriovenous malformation
    Carotid artery stenosis
    Venous hum
- Tumor
    Cerebellopontine angle tumors

Glomus tumors
Cerebral
Meningioma of middle ear
- Infection
Otitis media
- Trauma
Head trauma
After abnormally loud sounds

2.57 Tremors

Regular rhythmic trembling, usually in an extremity

Clinical Notes

Resting—occurs at rest
Action—three types
Intention—occurs with task-oriented movements
Contraction—occurs with isometric contraction
Postural—occurs during sustained maintenance of a
position

Differential Diagnosis

- Resting
Parkinson's disease
Hepatolenticular degeneration
Moderate to severe essential tremor
- Action
Physiologic (e.g., exaggerated by stress and anxiety)
Essential tremor
Primary writing tremor

Cerebellar tremor
Multiple sclerosis
Hepatolenticular degeneration
Hepatocerebral degeneration
Parkinson's disease
Drugs (e.g., caffeine, amphetamines, theophylline, ethanol)
Heavy metal poisoning

2.58 Vertigo

Illusion of movement of self or surroundings

Differential Diagnosis

- Miscellaneous
    Motion sickness
    Benign positional vertigo
    Drugs (e.g., alcohol, phenytoin, phenobarbital, salicylates, furosemide)
    Meniere's disease
    Arnold-Chiari malformation
    Syringobulbia
    Epilepsy (temporal lobe)
- Vascular
    Transient ischemic attack
    Cerebrovascular accident
    Cerebellar hemorrhage
- Tumors
    Posterior fossa

- Inflammation
    Labyrinthitis
    Vestibular neuritis
- Demyelination
    Multiple sclerosis

DIFFERENTIAL DIAGNOSIS BASED ON DIAGNOSTIC IMAGING

2.59 Extra-axial Posterior Fossa Masses in Children

Arachnoid cyst (m.c.)
Others are very rare

2.60 Common Extra-axial Posterior Fossa Masses in Adults

Acoustic neuroma (m.c.)
Meningioma
Epidermoid
Chordoma
Trigeminal neuroma

2.61 Intracranial Calcification

Differential Diagnosis

- Vascular
    Atherosclerosis (m.c.)
    Aneurysm
    Chronic subdural hematoma

      Arteriovenous malformation
- Infection
  - Abscess
  - Tuberculosis
  - Toxoplasmosis
  - Cytomegalovirus
  - Rubella
  - Cysticercosis
- Tumor
  - Glioma
  - Meningioma
  - Craniopharyngioma
  - Chordoma
- Metabolic/endocrine
  - Lead poisoning
  - Renal failure
  - Hypoparathyroidism

2.62 Intra-axial Cerebral Masses in Adults

Astrocytoma (m.c.) (e.g., Glioblastoma multiforme)
Metastasis
Oligodendroglioma
Arteriovenous malformation
Colloid cyst

2.63 Intra-axial Posterior Fossa Masses in Children

Medulloblastoma
Astrocytoma

Ependymomas
Brainstem glioma

2.64 Common Intra-axial Posterior Fossa Masses in Adults

Metastasis (m.c.)
Hemangioblastoma
Ependymoma
Cerebellar astrocytoma
Brainstem astrocytoma
Medulloblastoma

2.65 Intrasellar Masses

Pituitary adenoma (m.c.)
Fibroma
Angioma
Meningioma
Cholesteatoma
Teratoma

2.66 Intradural Extramedullary Spinal Cord Lesion

Neurofibroma (m.c.)
Neurinoma
Meningioma
Metastasis
Lipoma

2.67 Intradural Intramedullary Spinal Cord Lesion

Ependymoma (m.c.)
Astrocytoma
Hemangioblastoma
Metastasis

2.68 Extradural Spinal Lesions

Herniated nucleus pulposus (m.c.)
Metastasis
Lipoma
Bone tumors

2.69 Mass within the Third Ventricle

Differential Diagnosis

- Children
    Astrocytoma
    Neurofibromatosis
    Germinoma
    Histiocytosis X
    Glioma
    Craniopharyngioma
    Choroid plexus papilloma
    Ependymal cyst
    Vascular malformation
- Adults
    Colloid cyst (m.c.)
    Metastasis

Glioma
Vertebrobasilar ectasia/aneurysm
Meningioma

2.70 Mass within the Lateral Ventricle

Differential Diagnosis

- Children
   Ependymoma (m.c.)
   Choroid plexus papilloma
   Teratoma
   Astrocytoma
- Adult
   Astrocytoma (m.c.)
   Metastasis
   Meningioma
   Subependymoma
   Colloid cyst
   Lymphoma
   Neuroepithelial cyst

2.71 Mass within the Fourth Ventricle

Differential Diagnosis

- Children
   Ependymoma
   Medulloblastoma

Astrocytoma
Glioma
- Adults
  Choroid plexus papilloma (m.c.)
  Metastasis
  Epidermoid tumor
  Subependymoma

2.72 Common Causes of Cerebral Atrophy

Atherosclerotic dementia
Senile dementia
Alzheimer's disease
Chronic steroid therapy (reverses after cessation of therapy)

Chapter 3

Skeletal Disorders: Differential Diagnosis Based on Radiography

JOINT DISEASE

3.1 Ankylosis of Interphalangeal Joints

- Osseous ankylosis
  Ankylosing spondylitis (m.c.)
  Arthritis associated with psoriasis
  Erosive osteoarthritis
- Fibrous ankylosis
  Rheumatoid arthritis (m.c.)
  Still's disease

3.2 Arthritis with Osteopenia

- Inflammatory arthropathy
  Rheumatoid arthritis (m.c.)
  Reiter's syndrome (acute)
- Connective tissue arthropathy
  Progressive systemic sclerosis
  Systemic lupus erythematosus
- Infectious arthritis
- Miscellaneous
  Hemophilic arthropathy

3.3 Arthritis without Osteopenia

- Degenerative joint disease (m.c.)
- Inflammatory arthropathy
    Ankylosing spondylitis
    Arthritis associated with psoriasis
    Reiter's syndrome (long-standing)
    Arthritis associated with enteropathy
- Crystal deposition arthropathy
    Gouty arthritis
    Calcium pyrophosphate crystal deposition disease
- Miscellaneous
    Neuropathic arthropathy
    Pigmented villonodular synovitis

3.4 Arthritis with Periosteal Reaction

- Inflammatory arthropathy
    Juvenile chronic arthritis (m.c.)
    Arthritis associated with psoriasis
    Reiter's syndrome
- Infectious arthropathy
- Miscellaneous
    Hemophilic arthropathy

3.5 Arthropathy with Widened Joint Space

- Inflammatory arthropathy
    Rheumatoid arthritis (early) (m.c.)
    Arthritis associated with psoriasis

- Crystal deposition arthropathy
    Gouty arthritis
- Miscellaneous
    Pigmented villonodular synovitis
    Acromegaly

3.6 Axial Migration of the Femoral Head

- Inflammatory arthropathy
    Rheumatoid arthritis
    Ankylosing spondylitis
- Crystal deposition arthropathy
    Calcium pyrophosphate crystal deposition disease
- Infection
    Septic arthritis

3.7 Chondrocalcinosis

- Degenerative joint disease (m.c.)
- Crystal deposition arthropathy
    Gouty arthritis
    Calcium pyrophosphate crystal deposition disease
- Miscellaneous
    Idiopathic
    Hemophilic arthropathy
    Hepatolenticular degeneration (Wilson's disease)
    Ochronosis

3.8 Erosions with Preservation of Joint Space

- Miscellaneous
    Synovial chondrometaplasia (m.c.)
    Pigmented villonodular synovitis
- Hematologic
    Hemophilia
- Crystal deposition arthropathy
    Gouty arthritis

3.9 High-riding Humeral Head

- Soft tissue disease
    Rotator cuff tendinitis/tear (m.c.)
- Inflammatory arthropathy
    Rheumatoid arthritis
- Crystal deposition arthropathy
    Calcium pyrophosphate crystal deposition disease

3.10 Intra-articular Loose Bodies

- Degenerative joint disease (m.c.)
- Trauma
    Osteochondritis dissecans
    Avulsion fracture
- Miscellaneous
    Primary synovial chondrometaplasia
    Neuropathic arthropathy

3.11 Monarticular Arthropathy

- Degenerative joint disease (m.c.)
- Infectious arthritis
     Suppurative
     Tuberculous
- Trauma
     Post-traumatic synovitis (acute)
     Degenerative joint disease (chronic)
- Crystal deposition arthropathy
     Gouty arthritis
     Calcium pyrophosphate crystal deposition disease
- Miscellaneous
     Pigmented villonodular synovitis
     Sympathetic effusion

3.12 Premature Degenerative Joint Disease

- Trauma (m.c.)
- Miscellaneous
     Neuropathic arthropathy
     Acromegaly
     Hemophilic arthropathy
- Crystal deposition disease
     Calcium pyrophosphate crystal deposition disease

3.13 Protrusio Acetabuli

- Inflammatory arthropathy
     Rheumatoid arthritis (m.c.)
     Ankylosing spondylitis

- Miscellaneous
    Paget's disease
    Osteomalacia/osteoporosis
    Idiopathic
- Degenerative joint disease

3.14 Sacroilitis

- Bilaterally symmetric
    Ankylosing spondylitis (m.c.)
    Arthritis associated with enteropathy
    Hyperparathyroidism
- Bilateral but Asymmetric
    Arthritis associated with psoriasis
    Rheumatoid arthritis
- Unilateral
    Infectious arthritis
    Gouty arthritis

3.15 Cysts on Both Sides of a Joint

Degenerative joint disease (m.c.)
Pigmented villonodular synovitis
Calcium pyrophosphate deposition disease

3.16 Periarticular Calcification

- Arthritides
    Hydroxyapatite deposition disease (m.c.)
    Progressive systemic sclerosis

Gout
Calcium pyrophosphate deposition disease
Seronegative spondyloarthropathies
Synovial chondrometaplasia
- Metabolic/endocrine
    Hyperparathyroidism
    Diabetes mellitus
    Fluorosis
- Tumor
    Synovioma

BONE TUMORS

3.17 Age Incidence of Benign Bone Tumors

- Child
    Simple bone cyst
    Chondroblastoma
- Adolescent
    Fibroxanthoma
    Osteochondroma
    Osteoblastoma
    Enchondroma
- Adult
    Aneurysmal bone cyst
    Osteoid osteoma
    Chondromyxoid fibroma
    Osteoma

3.18 Age Incidence of Malignant Primary Bone Tumors

- Child
    Ewing's sarcoma
    Neuroblastoma
- Adolescent
    Osteosarcoma
- Adult
    Multiple myeloma
    Primary lymphoma of bone
    Chondrosarcoma
    Fibrosarcoma
    Osteosarcoma
    Chordoma
    Giant cell tumor

3.19 Cartilaginous Tumors of the Skeleton

- Benign
    Enchondroma
    Osteochondroma
    Chondromyxoid fibroma
    Chondroblastoma
- Malignant
    Chondrosarcoma

3.20 Central Medullary Lesion

- Benign
    Enchondroma
    Simple bone cyst

- Malignant
    Metastasis (m.c.)
    Multiple myeloma
    Primary lymphoma of bone

3.21 Cortical Lesion

- Benign
    Nonossifying fibroma
    Osteoid osteoma
- Malignant
    Metastasis (m.c.)
    Multiple myeloma

3.22 Diaphyseal Lesion

- Benign
    Nonossifying fibroma
    Solitary bone cyst (in adults)
    Enchondroma
- Malignant
    Metastasis (m.c.)
    Multiple myeloma
    Primary lymphoma of bone
    Ewing's sarcoma

3.23 Eccentric Medullary Lesion

- Benign
    Aneurysmal bone cyst
    Chondromyxoid fibroma

- Malignant
    Giant cell tumor
    Osteosarcoma
    Chondrosarcoma
    Fibrosarcoma

3.24 Epiphyseal Lesion

- Benign
    Subchrondral cyst of degenerative joint disease (m.c.)
    Intraosseous ganglion cyst
    Chondroblastoma
- Malignant
    Giant cell tumor

3.25 Fibrous Tumors of the Skeleton

- Benign
    Fibroxanthoma
    Chondromyxoid fibroma
- Malignant
    Fibrosarcoma
    Malignant fibrous histiocytoma

3.26 Juxtacortical Lesion

- Benign
    Juxtacortical chondroma
    Osteochondroma
- Malignant
    Parosteal osteosarcoma

3.27 Metaphyseal Lesion

- Benign
  Fibroxanthoma
  Solitary bone cyst
  Aneurysmal bone cyst
  Osteochondroma
  Chondromyxoid fibroma
- Malignant
  Metastasis (m.c.)
  Osteosarcoma
  Chondrosarcoma
  Fibrosarcoma
  Multiple myeloma

3.28 Osseous Tumors of the Skeleton

- Benign
  Enostoma (bone island)
  Osteoma
  Osteoid osteoma
- Malignant
  Osteosarcoma

3.29 Painful Scoliosis

- Benign
  Osteoid osteoma (m.c.)
  Aneurysmal bone cyst
  Osteoblastoma
  Fracture

- Malignant
  Giant cell tumor
  Metastasis

3.30 Subarticular Lesions

- Benign
  Subchondral cyst of degenerative joint disease (m.c.)
  Chondroblastoma
- Malignant
  Giant cell tumor

PERIOSTEAL REACTIONS

3.31 Laminated Periosteal Reaction (see also 5.6)

- Benign
  Osteomyelitis
  Callous formation
- Malignant
  Osteosarcoma
  Ewing's sarcoma

3.32 Periosteal Reaction in Children

- Benign
  Physiologic
  Battered child syndrome
  Caffey's disease (infantile cortical hyperostosis)
  Hypervitaminosis A

Osteogenesis imperfecta
Scurvy
- Malignant
  Acute leukemia
  Metastasis (neuroblastoma)
  Osteosarcoma
  Ewing's sarcoma

3.33 Solid Periosteal Reaction (see also 5.6)

- Benign
  Callous formation
  Osteoid osteoma
  Chronic osteomyelitis
  Hypertrophic osteoarthropathy
  Chronic vascular disease
- Malignant
  Low-grade malignancies

3.34 Spiculated Periosteal Reaction (see also 5.6)

- Benign
  Acute osteomyelitis
- Malignant
  Osteosarcoma
  Ewing's sarcoma
  Leukemia
  Chondrosarcoma
  Fibrosarcoma
  Metastasis

3.35 Symmetric Periosteal Reaction

- Benign
    Chronic vascular insufficiency
    Hypertrophic osteoarthropathy
    Thyroid acropachy

SKELETAL OPACIFICATION

3.36 Bone-within-a-Bone Appearance

- Metabolic/endocrine
    Acromegaly
    Paget's disease
- Vascular
    Sickle cell disease
    Thalassemia
- Dysplasias
    Osteopetrosis
- Physiologic
    Normal
- Miscellaneous
    Caffey's disease (Infantile cortical hyperostosis)
    Radiation

3.37 Diffuse Skeletal Sclerosis

- Tumors
    Diffuse blastic metastasis (m.c.)
    Multiple myeloma (3% of cases)
    Mastocytosis

- Metabolic/endocrine
    Secondary hyperparathyroidism
    Fluorosis
- Miscellaneous
    Myelosclerosis
- Dysplasias
    Osteopetrosis

3.38 Most Common Causes of Blastic Metastases

Breast carcinoma (m.c. in females)
Prostate carcinoma (m.c. in males)
Bronchogenic carcinoma
Lymphoma
Bladder carcinoma
Medulloblastoma
Colon carcinoma

3.39 Multiple Sclerotic Skeletal Lesions

- Tumor
    Blastic metastasis (m.c. malignant)
    Lymphoma
    Multiple osteomas
    Multiple myelomas (3% of cases)
- Congenital
    Osteopoikilosis (m.c. benign)
    Osteopathia striata
    Osteopetrosis

- Trauma
    Multiple fractures
    Battered child syndrome
- Miscellaneous
    Melorheostosis
    Paget's disease
- Vascular
    Medullary bone infarcts

3.40 Opaque Metaphyseal Bands

- Metabolic/endocrine
    Heavy metal poisoning
    Healing rickets
    Scurvy
    Cretinism
- Miscellaneous
    Normal variant (m.c. in infants)
    Systemic illness

3.41 Single Sclerotic Skeletal Lesion with Central Lucency

- Tumor
    Osteoid osteoma (m.c.)
    Osteoblastoma
- Infection
    Brodie's abscess

3.42 Single Sclerotic Skeletal Lesion

- Tumor
     Enostoma (m.c.)
     Metastasis
     Lymphoma
     Skeletal sarcomas
     Osteoma
     Osteoid osteoma
     Healing fibroxanthoma
     Osteoblastoma
- Trauma
     Callous
- Infection
     Brodie's abscess
     Sclerosing osteomyelitis
- Vascular
     Medullary bone infarct
     Avascular necrosis

3.43 Excess Callous Formation

- Metabolic/endocrine
     Steroid therapy (m.c.)
     Cushing's syndrome
     Secondary hyperparathyroidism
- Arthropathy
     Neuropathic arthropathy
- Trauma
     Battered child syndrome
     Nonaccidental injury (adults)

- Congenital
    Osteogenesis imperfecta

SKELETAL RAREFACTION

3.44 Acro-osteolysis

- Trauma
    Frostbite
    Burns
- Vascular
    Raynaud's disease
    Atherosclerosis
- Arthropathy
    Arthritis associated with psoriasis
    Progressive systemic sclerosis
    Neuropathic arthropathy
- Metabolic/endocrine
    Diabetes mellitus
    Hyperparathyroidism
- Miscellaneous
    Polyvinyl chloride exposure
    Sarcoidosis

3.45 Bubbly Bone Lesions

- Tumor
    Benign
        Fibroxanthoma
        Osteoblastoma

    Aneurysmal bone cyst
    Chondroblastoma
    Chondromyxoid fibroma
    Enchondroma
    Unicameral bone cyst
  Malignant
    Plasmacytoma
    Metastasis
    Giant cell tumor
- Infection
    Brodie's abscess
    Fungal infection

3.46 Diffuse Osteopenia

- Metabolic/endocrine
    Osteoporosis (m.c.)
    Osteomalacia
    Hyperparathyroidism
- Tumor
    Myeloma
    Metastasis

3.47 Diffuse Osteopenia in Children

- Tumor
    Leukemia (m.c.)
- Metabolic/endocrine
    Rickets
    Scurvy

       Secondary hyperparathyroidism
       Chronic hepatic disease
- Hematologic
       Anemias
- Dysplasias
       Osteogenesis imperfecta

3.48 Causes of Osteoporosis

- Metabolic/endocrine
       Postmenopausal (m.c.)
       Hyperthyroidism
       Hyperparathyroidism
       Acromegaly
       Addison's disease
       Malnutrition
       Chronic liver disease
       Malabsorption syndromes
       Diabetes mellitus
       Alcoholism
- Idiopathic
       Juvenile osteoporosis
       Adult osteoporosis
       Senile osteoporosis
       Transient osteoporosis of the hip
       Regional migratory osteoporosis
       Reflex sympathetic dystrophy
- Medications
       Heparin
       Corticosteroids

      Vitamin A
      Methotrexate
- Immobilization
- Arthropathy
      Rheumatoid arthritis
      Rheumatoid variants

3.49 Lucent Lesion with Surrounding Sclerosis

- Tumor
      Osteoid osteoma
      Osteoblastoma
- Trauma
      Stress fracture
- Infection
      Brodie's abscess

3.50 Lucent Metaphyseal Bands

- Tumor
      Leukemia
      Lymphoma
      Metastasis
- Miscellaneous
      Normal variant
      Severe illness
- Trauma
      Battered child syndrome
- Metabolic/endocrine
      Scurvy

3.51 Multicameral Geographic Nonexpansile Bone Lesion

- Tumor
    Aneurysmal bone cyst
    Solitary bone cyst
    Giant cell tumor
- Miscellaneous
    Fibrous dysplasia

3.52 Permeative Lesion without Periosteal Reaction

- Tumor
    Metastasis (m.c.)
    Myeloma
    Giant cell tumor
    Chondrosarcoma
    Telangiectatic osteosarcoma
    Hemangioma

3.53 Permeative Lesion with Periosteal Reaction

- Tumor
    Osteosarcoma (m.c.)
    Ewing's sarcoma
    Fibrosarcoma
- Infection
    Acute osteomyelitis

3.54 Regional/Localized Osteopenia

- Miscellaneous
    Disuse atrophy of bone (m.c.)
    Transient osteoporosis of the hip
    Regional migratory osteoporosis
- Trauma
    Post-traumatic osteolysis
    Reflex sympathetic dystrophy syndrome
- Arthropathy
    Rheumatoid arthritis
    Systemic lupus erythematosus

3.55 Rib Lesions

- Tumor
    Metastasis (m.c. malignant lesion)
    Myeloma
    Chondrosarcoma
    Ewing's sarcoma
    Enchondroma
    Osteochondroma
    Eosinophilic granuloma
- Miscellaneous
    Fibrous dysplasia (m.c. benign lesion)
    Callous formation
    Paget's disease
    Brown tumor
- Infection
    Osteomyelitis

3.56 Unicameral Geographic Nonexpansile Bone Lesion

- Tumor
    Fibroxanthoma
    Giant cell tumor
    Enchondroma
    Simple bone cyst
    Metastasis
    Eosinophilic granuloma
- Trauma
    Post-traumatic ganglion cyst
    Epidermoid inclusion cyst
- Infection
    Osteomyelitis
- Metabolic/endocrine
    Brown tumor
- Arthropathy
    Subchondral cyst of degenerative joint disease
- Vascular
    Hemophilic pseudotumor
- Miscellaneous
    Fibrous dysplasia

3.57 Unicameral Geographic Expansile Bone Lesion

- Tumor
    Simple bone cyst
    Enchondroma
    Aneurysmal bone cyst
    Fibroxanthoma

Eosinophilic granuloma
Giant cell tumor (benign form)
Chordoma
Plasmacytoma
- Metabolic/endocrine
Brown tumor

3.58 Vertebral Body Striations

- Metabolic/endocrine
Osteoporosis (m.c.)
- Tumor
Hemangioma
- Miscellaneous
Paget's disease

SKULL

3.59 "Hair on End" Cranial Vault

- Hematologic
Sickle cell disease (m.c.)
Thalassemia
Iron-deficiency anemia
- Tumor
Hemangioma
Meningioma
Plasmacytoma
Metastasis (neuroblastoma)

3.60 Basilar Invagination

- Congenital
  Platybasia
  Atlanto-occipital assimilation
  Klippel-Feil syndrome
  Osteogenesis imperfecta
  Achondroplasia
  Cleidocranial dysplasia

- Metabolic/endocrine
  Rickets

- Miscellaneous
  Paget's disease
  Fibrous dysplasia

3.61 Button Sequestrum

- Tumor
  Metastasis
  Eosinophilic granuloma
  Epidermoid tumor

- Infection
  Tuberculosis
  Osteomyelitis

- Miscellaneous
  Radiation therapy

3.62 Destruction of the Clivus

- Tumor
    Chordoma
    Metastasis
- Infection
    Osteomyelitis

3.63 Enlarged Sella Turcica

- Tumor
    Pituitary adenoma (chromophobe adenoma m.c.)
    Craniopharyngioma
    Prolactinoma
    Meningioma
- Vascular
    Carotid artery aneurysm
- Miscellaneous
    Increased intracranial pressure
    Empty sella syndrome

3.64 Increased Opacity of Skull Base

- Miscellaneous
    Fibrous dysplasia (m.c.)
    Paget's disease
- Tumor
    Metastasis
    Meningioma

- Infection
    Chronic otitis media
    Mastoiditis

3.65 Lucent Cranial Lesion(s)

- Tumor
    Myeloma (m.c.)
    Metastasis
    Histiocytosis X
    Hemangioma
    Epidermoid tumor
- Infection
    Osteomyelitis
    Tuberculosis
- Trauma
    Leptomeningeal cyst
    Surgical burr hole
- Metabolic/endocrine
    Hyperparathyroidism
- Miscellaneous
    Sarcoidosis
    Paget's disease (osteoporosis circumscripta)
    Radiation therapy

3.66 Sclerotic Cranial Lesion(s)

- Tumor
    Metastasis (m.c.)
    Myeloma

       Osteoma (especially in sinuses)
       Meningioma (causes localized sclerosis)
- Miscellaneous
       Paget's disease
       Fibrous dysplasia
       Hyperostosis frontalis interna
       Brown tumor (treated)

3.67 Small Sella Turcica

- Miscellaneous
       Normal variant (m.c.)
       Radiation therapy
- Metabolic/endocrine
       Hypopituitarism

3.68 Widened Sutures

- Miscellaneous
       Hydrocephalus (m.c.)
- Tumor
       Brain tumors (with increased intracranial pressure)
       Neuroblastoma
       Leukemia
       Lymphoma
- Metabolic/endocrine
       Rickets
       Secondary hyperparathyroidism

SPINAL LESIONS

3.69 Erosion/Absence of a Pedicle

- Tumor
    Metastasis (m.c.)
    Myeloma (late)
    Aneurysmal bone cyst
    Osteoblastoma
- Congenital
    Aplasia
- Infection
    Tuberculosis

3.70 Anterior Scalloping of a Vertebra

- Vascular
    Abdominal aortic aneurysm (m.c.)
- Tumor
    Retroperitoneal lymphoma
    Lymphadenopathy
- Infection
    Tuberculosis

3.71 Atlantoaxial Instability

- Trauma (m.c.)
    Transverse ligament rupture
    Type II odontoid fracture

- Arthropathy
  Rheumatoid arthritis
  Seronegative spondyloarthropathies
  Juvenile chronic arthritis
  Systemic lupus erythematosus
- Congenital
  Trisomy 21
  Odontoid hypoplasia
  Os odontoideum
  Atlanto-occipital assimilation
- Infection
  Retropharyngeal abscess
  Grisel's syndrome

3.72 Block Vertebra

- Congenital
  Single congenital (m.c.)
  Klippel-Feil syndrome
- Arthropathy
  Rheumatoid arthritis
  Ankylosing spondylitis
- Surgical
  Arthrodesis
- Trauma
  Post-traumatic
- Infection
  Tuberculosis

3.73 Calcification of Disc(s)

- Arthropathy
    Degenerative disc disease (m.c.)
    Calcium pyrophosphate crystal deposition disease
    Ankylosing spondylitis
    Juvenile chronic arthritis
    Gouty arthritis
    Diffuse idiopathic skeletal hyperostosis
- Metabolic/endocrine
    Ochronosis
    Hemochromatosis
- Idiopathic

3.74 Opaque Vertebral Pedicle

- Tumor
    Metastasis (m.c.)
    Osteoid osteoma
    Osteoblastoma
- Trauma
    Secondary to contralateral spondylolysis
- Congenital
    Secondary to absence of contralateral pedicle

3.75 Enlarged Vertebral Body

- Miscellaneous
    Paget's disease (m.c.)

- Metabolic/endocrine
    Acromegaly
    Gigantism
- Tumor
    Giant cell tumor
    Aneurysmal bone cyst
    Hemangioma
- Infection
    Hydatid disease

3.76 Enlarged Neural Foramen

- Tumor
    Neurofibroma (m.c.)
    Intracanalicular mass
- Congenital
    Pedicle aplasia
    Dural ectasia
- Vascular
    Erosion by tortuous vertebral artery

3.77 Homogenously Sclerotic Vertebra

- Tumor
    Metastasis (m.c.)
    Lymphoma
- Miscellaneous
    Paget's disease
- Infection
    Chronic, low grade

3.78 Hypoplastic Vertebral Body

- Congenital
  Block vertebra (m.c.)
  Gaucher's disease
- Arthropathy
  Juvenile chronic arthritis
- Miscellaneous
  Radiation therapy

3.79 Multiple Collapsed Vertebra

- Miscellaneous
  Osteoporosis (m.c.)
- Tumor
  Metastasis
  Myeloma
- Trauma
  Compression fractures
  Scheuermann's disease
- Infection
  Tuberculosis

3.80 "Phytes" of the Spine (Figure 3-1)

- Osteophytes
  Degenerative disc disease (m.c.)
  Stress from hypermobility
- Syndesmophytes
  Ankylosing spondylitis (m.c.)
  Ochronosis

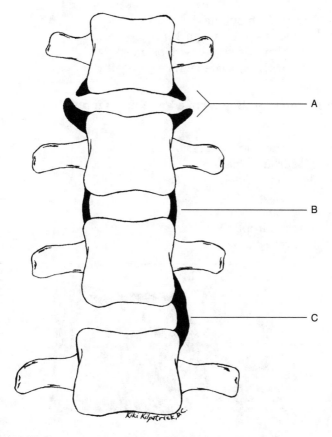

Note: (A) osteophytes; (B) syndesmophyte; (C) parasyndesmophyte.

Figure 3-1 "Phytes" of the Spine. *Source:* Copyright © 1993 by Kiki Kilpatrick, D.C.

- Parasyndesmophytes
  Reiter's syndrome (m.c.)
  Arthritis associated with psoriasis
  Arthritis associated with enteropathy

3.81 Posterior Scalloping of a Vertebra (Figure 3-2)

- Tumors
  Intracanalicular mass (m.c.)
  Neurofibromatosis
- Metabolic/endocrine
  Acromegaly
- Congenital
  Achondroplasia
  Dural ectasia

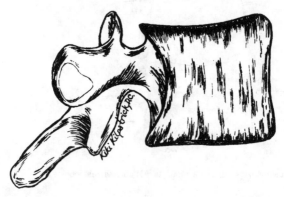

Figure 3-2 Posterior Vertebral Body Scalloping. *Source:* Copyright © 1993 by Kiki Kilpatrick, D.C.

- Miscellaneous
    Hydrocephalus (communicating type)
    Syringohydromyelia

3.82 Single Collapsed Vertebra

- Tumor
    Metastasis (m.c. for pathologic collapse)
    Myeloma
    Giant cell tumor
    Hemangioma (rare)
    Eosinophilic granuloma
    Aneurysmal bone cyst
- Trauma
    Compression fracture (m.c. for nonpathologic collapse)
- Miscellaneous
    Osteoporosis
- Infection
    Tuberculosis

3.83 Squaring of a Vertebra

- Arthropathy
    Ankylosing spondylitis (m.c.)
    Arthritis associated with psoriasis
    Reiter's syndrome
    Rheumatoid arthritis
- Miscellaneous
    Paget's disease

3.84 Vacuum Phenomenon

- Arthropathy
  Degenerative disc disease (m.c.)
- Trauma
  Schmorl's node
  Disc injury (vacuum cleft sign)
- Tumor
  Metastasis with collapsed vertebra

3.85 Vertebral Endplate Irregularity

- Trauma
  Schmorl's node (m.c.)
  Limbus bone
  Infractions (osteoporosis)
- Hematologic
  Sickle cell disease

3.86 Widened Interpediculate Distance

- Congenital
  Meningiomyelocele (m.c.)
  Diastematomyelia
- Tumor
  Intracanalicular mass

Part II

Helpful Lists

Chapter 4

Helpful Neurologic Lists

4.1 Anatomic Location of Lesions by Common Neurologic Signs

- Anterior spinal cord (Figure 4-1)
    Bilateral paresis
    Loss of pain and temperature
    Preservation of vibration and proprioception
- Brainstem
    Hemiparesis
    Contralateral cranial nerve findings
- Cauda equina
    Saddle anesthesia
    Bilateral leg pain (often asymmetric)
    Loss of bowel and bladder control
    Sexual dysfunction (e.g., loss of morning erections)
- Central spinal cord (e.g., syringomyelia) (Figure 4-2)
    Bilateral loss of pain and temperature
    Lower motor neuron signs at level of lesion
- Cerebellum
    Dysmetria
    Dysdiadochokinesia
    Ataxia

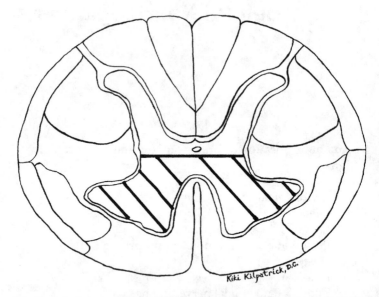

Figure 4-1 Anterior Spinal Cord Lesion. *Source:* Copyright © 1993 Kiki Kilpatrick, D.C.

    Intention tremor
    Hypotonia during passive movements
• Cerebral hemisphere
    Hemiparesis
    Facial weakness
    Hemisensory loss
    Aphasia
• Hemicord syndrome (Figure 4-3)
    Hemiparesis

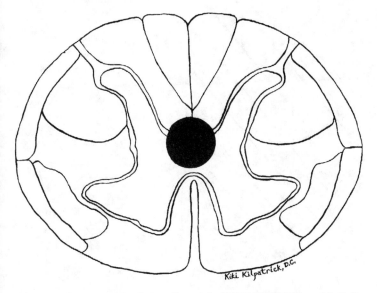

Figure 4-2 Syringomyelia. *Source:* Copyright © 1993 by Kiki Kilpatrick, D.C.

Contralateral loss of pain and temperature
Ipsilateral loss of vibration and proprioception
- Nerve root
    Dermatomal sensory loss
    Paresis/atrophy of muscle group innervated by
        specific nerve
    Atrophy of muscle group innervated by specific nerve
    Fasciculations
    Back/neck pain common

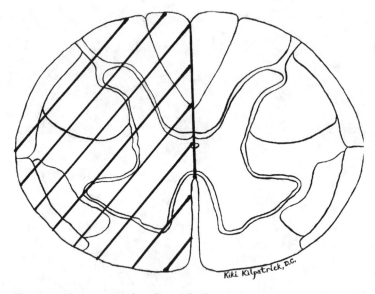

Figure 4-3 Hemisection of the Spinal Cord. *Source:* Copyright © 1993 by Kiki Kilpatrick, D.C.

- Neuromuscular junction
    Bilateral proximal limb paresis
    No sensory symptoms
- Peripheral nerve
    Paresis/atrophy of muscle group supplied by the
        nerve

Sensory loss in distribution supplied by nerve
Fasciculations
Back/neck pain uncommon
- Posterior spinal cord (Figure 4-4)
  Bilateral loss of vibration and proprioception

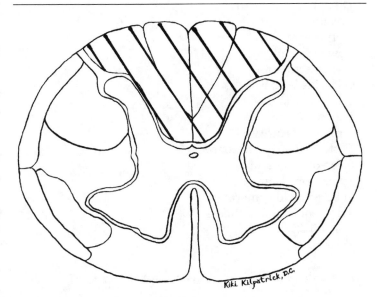

Figure 4-4 Posterior Spinal Cord Lesion. *Source:* Copyright © 1993 by Kiki Kilpatrick, D.C.

4.2 Most Common Neurologic Diseases (listed alphabetically)

Alcoholism
Benign brain tumors
Brain injury
Cerebral palsy
Cerebrovascular disease (acute)
Congenital malformations
Dementia
Disc protrusion/extrusion
Epilepsy
Herpes zoster
Low back pain
Meniere's disease
Migraine headache
Multiple sclerosis
Neck pain
Parkinson's disease
Postconcussive syndromes
Sleep disorders
Spinal cord injury
Subarachnoid hemorrhage
Transient ischemic attacks
Trisomy 21
Tumors

4.3 Vascular Brain Diseases (listed alphabetically)

Abnormal coagulation
Aneurysm

Arteriovenous fistula
Arteriovenous malformation
Atherosclerosis
Cavernous angioma
Cerebrovascular accident
Connective tissue diseases with vasculitis
Hemangioma
Hematoma
Migraine headache
Small vessel vasculitides
Subarachnoid hemorrhage
Thromboembolism
Transient ischemic attack
Venous angioma

4.4 Signs and Symptoms of Occlusive Cerebrovascular Disease by Location

Artery	Signs/Symptoms
Anterior cerebral	Urinary incontinence
	Upper motor neuron lesion signs
	Leg affected worse than arm
Middle cerebral	Homonymous hemianopia
	Upper motor neuron lesion signs
	Face and arm worse than leg
	Sensory loss
	Aphasia
Posterior cerebral	Homonymous hemianopia
	Hemianesthesia

4.5 Brain Tumors and Tumor-like Lesions (listed alphabetically by location)

- Brainstem
    Astrocytoma (m.c.)
    Metastasis
    Venous angioma
- Cerebellopontine angle
    Acoustic neuroma (m.c.)
    Arachnoid cyst
    Choroid plexus papilloma
    Cranial nerves V, VII, IX, X, XI, XII neuromas
    Ependymoma
    Epidermoid cyst
    Meningioma
    Metastasis
    Paraganglioma
- Cerebellum
    Medulloblastoma (m.c. in children)
    Metastasis (m.c. in adults)
    Astrocytoma
    Cavernous angioma
    Hemangioblastoma
- Cerebral hemisphere
    Glioblastoma multiforme (m.c.)
    Astrocytoma
    Cavernous angioma
    Ependymoma
    Meningioma
    Metastasis

Oligodendroglioma
Primary central nervous system lymphoma

- Corpus callosum
  Astrocytoma
  Glioblastoma multiforme
  Lipoma
  Metastasis
  Oligodendroglioma
- Fourth ventricle
  Choroid plexus papilloma (m.c.)
  Ependymoma
  Meningioma
  Subependymoma
- Optic nerve/chiasm
  Meningioma (m.c.)
  Astrocytoma
- Pineal gland
  Germinoma (m.c.)
  Epidermoid cyst
  Pinealoma
  Teratoma (benign and malignant)
- Sella turcica region
  Craniopharyngioma (m.c. suprasellar mass)
  Pituitary adenoma (m.c. intrasellar mass)
  Dermoid cyst
  Germinoma
  Meningioma
- Third ventricle
  Colloid cyst (m.c.)
  Astrocytoma

Ependymoma
Metastasis
Oligodendroglioma

4.6 Spinal Cord Tumors

- Intradural/extramedullary
  Schwannoma (m.c.)
  Meningioma
  Neurofibroma
- Intradural/intramedullary
  Ependymoma (m.c.)
  Astrocytoma
  Glioblastoma

4.7 Most Common Metastasis to the Central Nervous System

Breast
Gastrointestinal tract
Kidney
Lung
Melanoma
Thyroid

4.8 Infectious Diseases of the Nervous System (listed alphabetically)

- Bacterial
  Meningococcus
  Mycobacterium

  Pneumococcus
  Staphylococcus
  Streptococcus
- Fungal
  Aspergillus
  Candida
  Cryptococcus
  Nocardia
- Parasites
  Echinococcus
  Toxoplasmosis
  Trichinosis
- Spirochetes
  Lyme disease
  Syphilis
- Viral
  Adenovirus
  Arbovirus
  Herpesvirus
  Human immunodeficiency virus
  Influenza
  Measles
  Mumps
  Poliovirus
  Rabies
  Varicella zoster

4.9 Common Demyelinating Diseases of the Nervous System

Multiple sclerosis
Leukodystrophies
Postinfectious demyelination

4.10 Most Common Congenital Malformations of the Nervous System

Arnold-Chiari malformation (Figure 4-5)
Basilar invagination
Dandy-Walker malformation
Neurofibromatosis

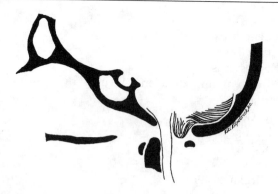

Note: herniation of cerebellar tonsils through foramen magnum.

Figure 4-5 Midsagittal Schematic of Type I Arnold-Chiari Malformation. *Source:* Copyright © 1993 by Kiki Kilpatrick, D.C.

4.11 Common Neurodegenerative Diseases of the Nervous System

Alzheimer's disease
Parkinson's disease

4.12 Cranial Foramina Contents (Figure 4-6)

- Carotid canal
    Carotid artery
    Sympathetic plexus
- Cribriform plate
    Cranial nerve I
    Ethmoidal arteries
- Foramen lacerum
    Meningeal branches of ascending pharyngeal artery
- Foramen magnum
    Medulla oblongata
    Cranial nerve XI (spinal segment)
    Vertebral arteries and veins
    Spinal arteries
- Foramen ovale
    Cranial nerve V (mandibular division)
    Lesser petrosal nerve
- Foramen rotundum
    Cranial nerve V (maxillary division)
- Foramen spinosum
    Middle meningeal artery
- Hypoglossal canal
    Cranial nerve XII

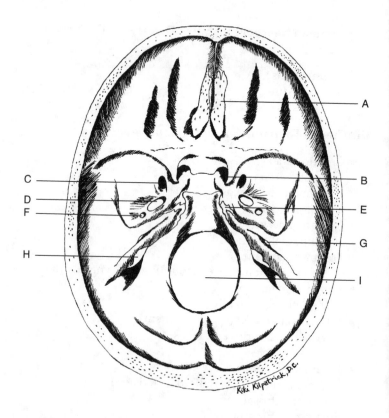

Note: (A) cribriform plate; (B) optic canal; (C) foramen rotundum; (D) foramen ovale; (E) foramen lacerum; (F) foramen spinosum; (G) internal acoustic meatus; (H) jugular foramen; (I) foramen magnum.

Figure 4-6 Foramen of the Base of the Skull. *Source:* Copyright © 1993 by Kiki Kilpatrick, D.C.

- Jugular foramen
    Cranial nerves IX, X, XI
    Internal jugular vein
    Inferior petrosal sinus
- Optic canal
    Cranial nerve II
    Ophthalmic artery
- Stylomastoid foramen
    Cranial nerve VII
- Superior orbital fissure
    Cranial nerves III, IV, VI, and V (ophthalmic division)

4.13 Major Spinal Cord Tracts and Their Function (Figure 4-7)

- Corticospinal
    Primary motor pathway
- Lateral spinothalamic
    Pain
    Temperature
    Gross touch
- Posterior columns
    Vibration
    Proprioception
    Fine touch
- Anterior/posterior spinocerebellar
    Coordination of motor activity

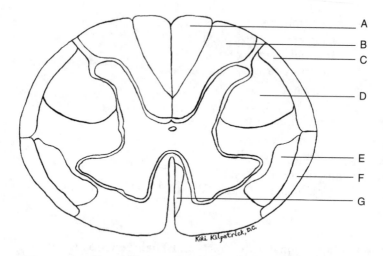

Note: (A) fasiculus gracilis; (B) fasiculus cuneatus; (C) posterior spinocerebellar tract; (D) lateral corticospinal tract; (E) lateral spinothalamic tract; (F) anterior spinocerebellar tract; (G) anterior corticospinal tract.

Figure 4-7 Cross Section of Adult Spinal Cord. *Source:* Copyright © 1993 by Kiki Kilpatrick, D.C.

4.14 Extrapyramidal (Basal Ganglia/Cerebellum) Syndromes

Parkinson's disease (m.c.)
Chorea
Athetosis
Hemiballismus
Dystonias
Hepatolenticular degeneration (Wilson's disease)

4.15 Neuroectodermal Syndromes (Phakomatoses)

Neurofibromatosis (m.c.)
Tuberous sclerosis
von Hippel-Lindau disease
Sturge-Weber disease (encephalotrigeminal angiomatosis)

4.16 Common Peripheral Nerve Entrapment Sites

Nerve	Entrapment Site
Brachial plexus	Thoracic outlet
Median	Carpal tunnel
Ulnar	Tunnel of Guyon
Peroneal	Fibular head
	Tarsal tunnel

4.17 Causes of Carpal Tunnel Syndrome

- Trauma
    Occupational microtrauma (m.c.)
    Post-traumatic deformity
- Metabolic/endocrine
    Diabetes mellitus
    Acromegaly
    Hypothyroidism
- Arthritides
    Rheumatoid arthritis
- Miscellaneous
    Pregnancy
    Obesity
    Idiopathic

4.18 Signs and Symptoms of Brachial Plexus Lesions

Location	Signs/Symptoms
Entire plexus	Lower motor neuron lesion in entire arm
	Sensory loss in entire arm
	Horner's syndrome
Upper plexus (Erb Duchenne palsy)	Loss of shoulder motion
	Loss of elbow flexion
	Sensory loss over lateral arm
Lower plexus (Klumpke's palsy)	Claw hand deformity
	Paralysis of intrinsic hand muscles
	Sensory loss over medial forearm/hand
	Horner's syndrome

4.19 Deep Tendon Reflexes (primary innervation in bold print)

Reflex	Innervation
Jaw jerk	**Cranial nerve V**
Biceps	C**5**, 6
Brachioradialis	C5, **6**
Pectoralis major	C5, **6**, 7
Triceps	C6, **7**, 8
Adductor	L2, **3**, 4
Knee jerk	L2, 3, **4**
Anterior tibialis	L4, **5**
Hamstring	L5, **S1**, 2
Achilles	L5, **S1**, 2

4.20 Superficial Reflexes

Reflex	Innervation
Corneal	Cranial nerve V (afferent), VII (efferent)
Pharyngeal (gag)	Cranial nerve IX (afferent), X (efferent)
Upper abdominal	T6–9
Middle abdominal	T9–11
Lower abdominal	T11–L1
Cremasteric	L1, 2
Anal	S3, 4, 5
Bulbocavernous	S3, 4

4.21 Pathologic Reflexes (indicate upper motor neuron lesion)

Babinski's reflex
Hoffmann's sign
Ankle clonus
Oppenheim's sign
Pronator drift

4.22 Common Cervical Nerve Root Syndromes

- C5
    Pain—C5 dermatome
    Hypoesthesia—C5 dermatome
    Hyporeflexia—biceps reflex
    Weakness—biceps, deltoid, supra/infraspinatus
- C6
    Pain—C6 dermatome
    Hypoesthesia—C6 dermatome

       Hyporeflexia—brachioradialis and pectoralis major
          reflexes
       Weakness—brachioradialis, pectoralis major

- C7

       Pain—C7 dermatome
       Hypoesthesia—C7 dermatome
       Hyporeflexia—triceps reflex
       Weakness—triceps, wrist extensors

- C8

       Pain—C8 dermatome
       Hypoesthesia—C8 dermatome
       Hyporeflexia—triceps possibly
       Weakness—intrinsic hand muscles

4.23 Common Lumbar Nerve Root Syndromes

- L4

       Pain—L4 dermatome
       Hypoesthesia—L4 dermatome
       Hyporeflexia—knee jerk
       Weakness—quadriceps muscle group

- L5

       Pain—L5 dermatome
       Hypoesthesia—L5 dermatome
       Hyporeflexia—anterior tibialis
       Weakness—Peroneus, toe extensors, anterior tibialis

- S1

       Pain—S1 dermatome
       Hypoesthesia—S1 dermatome
       Hyporeflexia—Achilles

Weakness—hamstring muscle group, plantar flexors, gluteus maximus

4.24 Upper versus Lower Motor Neuron Lesions

Sign	Upper	Lower
Paralysis	Spastic	Flaccid
Deep tendon reflexes	Increased	Decreased
Atrophy	+/–	+
Pathologic reflexes	+	–
Fasciculations	–	+

4.25 Brain versus Spinal Cord Lesion

Brain	Spinal Cord
Pathologic reflexes	Pathologic reflexes
Increased deep tendon reflexes	Increased deep tendon reflexes
Cranial nerve deficits	Dermatomal deficits
Ipsilateral sensory loss	Dissociation of sensory function

4.26 Intramedullary versus Extramedullary Spinal Cord Lesions

Signs	Intramedullary	Extramedullary
Nerve root pain	Rare	Common
Upper motor neuron lesion signs	Late onset	Early onset
Lower motor neuron lesion signs	Over many segments	Localized
Dissociation of sensation	Present	Rare

4.27 Signs of Spinal Cord Compression by Location

Region	Signs
Upper cervical	Upper motor neuron lesion signs in upper and lower extremities
	Loss of bowel and bladder control
Midcervical	Weakness of rhomboids, deltoids, biceps, brachioradialis
	Upper motor neuron lesion signs in rest of upper and all of lower extremities
	Loss of biceps reflex
	Loss of bowel and bladder control
Cervicothoracic	Weakness of intrinsic hand muscles
	Upper motor neuron lesion signs in lower extremities
	Loss of bowel and bladder control
Midthoracic	Intercostal muscle paralysis
	Upper motor neuron lesion signs in lower extremities
	Loss of upper abdominal reflexes
	Loss of bowel and bladder control
Lower thoracic	Loss of lower abdominal reflexes
	Cephalic migration of umbilicus
	Upper motor neuron lesion signs in lower extremities
	Loss of bowel and bladder control
Upper lumbar	Normal abdominal reflexes
	Loss of cremasteric reflex
	Upper motor neuron lesion signs in lower extremities
	Loss of bowel and bladder control
Cauda equina	Weakness in lower extremities
	Loss of knee jerk and Achille's reflex
	Upper motor neuron lesion signs in lower extremities
	Sensory loss in lower extremities
	Loss of bowel and bladder control
Sacral	Loss of anal reflex
	Saddle anesthesia
	Normal lower extremities

4.28 Types of Abnormal Sensation by Lesion Location

Location	Sensory Loss
Thalamus/upper brainstem	Total unilateral loss of all sensation
Lateral medulla	Ipsilateral pain and temperature loss on face
	Contralateral pain and temperature loss on body
Entire spinal cord	Bilateral loss of sensation below a specific level
One side of spinal cord	Ipsilateral loss of sensation below a specific level
Central spinal cord	Loss of pain and temperature over several segments
	Normal sensation above and below lesion
Posterior columns	Loss of position and vibration sense only
Nerve root	Dermatomal loss of sensation

4.29 Intracranial Pain–sensitive Structures

Basal dura
Pia mater
Venous sinuses and tributaries
Circle of Willis (Figure 4-8)
Nerves with sensory afferents

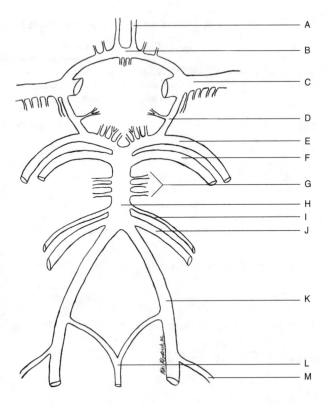

Note: (A) anterior cerebral artery; (B) anterior communicating artery; (C) middle cerebral artery; (D) posterior communicating artery; (E) posterior cerebral artery; (F) superior cerebellar artery; (G) pontine arteries; (H) basilar artery; (I) labyrinthine artery; (J) anterior inferior cerebellar artery; (K) vertebral artery; (L) anterior spinal artery; (M) posterior inferior cerebellar artery.

Figure 4-8 Circle of Willis. *Source:* Copyright © 1993 by Kiki Kilpatrick, D.C.

4.30 Signs and Symptoms of Cerebral Disease by Location

Lobe	Signs/Symptoms
Frontal	Personality change
	Primitive reflexes (e.g., grasp reflex)
	Ansomia
	Optic nerve atrophy
	Leg weakness
	Loss of bladder control
	Expressive aphasia
	Seizures
Temporal	Memory loss
	Receptive aphasia
	Upper quadrant hemianopia
	Seizures
Parietal	Aphasia
	Agraphia
	Acalculia
	Left-right disorientation
	Astereognosis
	Lower quadrant hemianopia
	Seizures
Occipital	Homonymous hemianopia
	Seizures

Chapter 5

Helpful Skeletal Radiology Lists

5.1 Most Common Skeletal Lesions by Category

Category	*Most Common Lesion*
Skeletal malignancy	Lytic metastasis
Primary skeletal malignancy	Multiple myeloma
Metastatic tumor to bone	Bronchogenic carcinoma
Benign tumor of bone	Bone island
Benign tumor of the spine	Hemangioma
Cause of osteopenia	Osteoporosis
Arthritis	Degenerative joint disease
Inflammatory arthritis	Rheumatoid arthritis
Spinal inflammatory arthritis	Ankylosing spondylitis
Fracture plane in adults	Oblique
Fractured bone in the body	Clavicle
Fracture of the spine	Simple compression fracture
Fractured bone in the wrist	Scaphoid
Fracture of the elbow	Radial head
Fracture of the hip	Subcapital region
Stress fracture	Second and third metatarsals
Shoulder dislocation	Anterior inferior
Dislocated bone in the wrist	Lunate
Hip dislocation	Posterior
Osteochondritis dissecans	Medial femoral condyle

5.2 Classification of Tumors

- Cartilaginous
    Benign
      Chondroblastoma
      Osteochondroma
      Enchondroma
      Chondromyxoid fibroma
    Malignant
      Chondrosarcoma
- Fibrous
    Benign
      Fibroxanthoma
    Malignant
      Fibrosarcoma
      Malignant fibrous histiocytoma
- Osseous
    Benign
      Enostoma
      Osteoma
      Osteoid osteoma
      Osteoblastoma
    Malignant
      Osteosarcoma and variants
- Round cell tumors
    Malignant
      Multiple myeloma
      Leukemia
      Primary lymphoma of bone (a.k.a. reticulum cell sarcoma)
      Ewing's sarcoma

- Miscellaneous
    - *Benign*
        - Aneurysmal bone cyst
        - Solitary bone cyst
        - Hemangioma
    - *Malignant*
        - Giant cell tumor
        - Chordoma

5.3 Most Common Bone Tumor Locations

Tumor	Location
Aneurysmal bone cyst	Femur
Bone island	Pelvis
Chondroblastoma	Humerus
Chondromyxoid fibroma	Tibia
Chondrosarcoma	Pelvis
Chordoma	Sacrum
Enchondroma	Metacarpal
Ewing's sarcoma	Pelvis
Fibrosarcoma	Femur
Fibroxanthoma	Femur
Giant cell tumor	Femur
Hemangioma	Spine
Metastasis	Spine
Multiple myeloma	Spine
Osteoblastoma	Femur
Osteochondroma	Femur
Osteoid osteoma	Femur
Osteoma	Skull
Osteosarcoma	Femur
Reticulum cell sarcoma	Femur
Solitary bone cyst	Humerus

5.4 Regional Bone Tumor Location

Region	Malignant	Benign
Diaphyseal	Ewing's sarcoma Metastasis Reticulum cell sarcoma Multiple myeloma	Osteoid osteoma Solitary bone cyst (late)
Metaphyseal	Metastasis Osteosarcoma Chondrosarcoma Fibrosarcoma	Bone island Osteochondroma Fibroxanthoma Osteoid osteoma Enchondroma Solitary bone cyst
Epiphyseal	Giant cell tumor	Chondroblastoma

5.5 Patterns of Bone Destruction (Figure 5-1)

Pattern	Description	Significance
Geographic	Solitary, well-defined	Benign, nonaggressive
Moth-eaten	Multiple, poorly defined	Aggressive, malignant
Permeative	Pinhead size, poorly defined	Aggressive, malignant

5.6 Types of Periosteal Reactions (Figure 5-2)

Type	Description	Significance
Solid	Thick, single layer	Benign, nonaggressive
Laminated	Thin, multilayered	Aggressive, malignant
Spiculated	Thin spicules, radiating	Aggressive, malignant

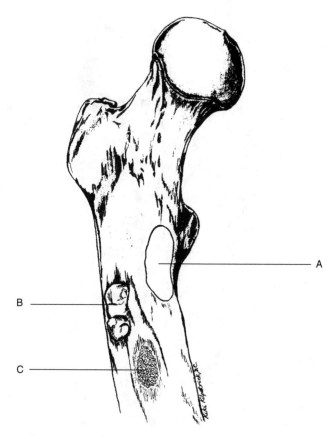

Note: (A) geographic; (B) moth-eaten; (C) permeative.

Figure 5-1 Typical Patterns of Bone Destruction. *Source:* Copyright © 1993 by Kiki Kilpatrick, D.C.

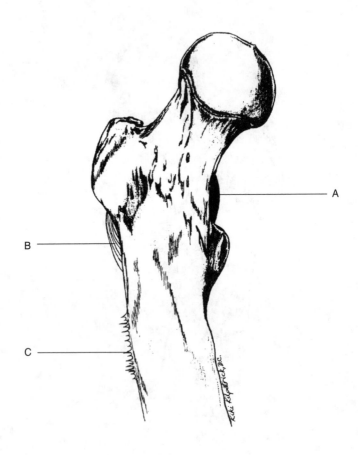

Note: (A) solid; (B) laminated; (C) spiculated.

Figure 5-2 Periosteal Reactions. *Source:* Copyright © 1993 by Kiki Kilpatrick, D.C.

5.7 Benign versus Malignant Bone Lesions

Sign	Benign	Malignant
Size	Small	Large
Sclerotic rim	Present	Absent or thin
Periosteal reaction	Solid	Laminated, spiculated
Soft tissue mass	Absent	Present
Cortical destruction	Absent	Present
Bone scan	Negative (usually)	Positive

5.8 Primary Malignancies Metastasizing to Bone and Their Appearance

Primary Tumor	Radiographic Appearance
Lung	Lytic
Breast	Lytic, blastic, mixed
Prostate	Blastic
Thyroid	Lytic
Renal	Lytic
Bladder	Lytic
Colon	Lytic
Stomach	Blastic
Melanoma	Lytic
Cervix	Lytic
Gonads	Lytic

5.9 Tumors of the Spine

- Benign
  Hemangioma (m.c.)
  Osteoid osteoma

Osteoblastoma
Aneurysmal bone cyst
- Malignant
Metastasis (m.c.)
Multiple myeloma
Giant cell tumor
Leukemia
Lymphoma

5.10 Classification of Common Arthritides

- Inflammatory
Rheumatoid arthritis (m.c.)
Ankylosing spondylitis
Reiter's syndrome
Arthritis associated with psoriasis
Arthritis associated with enteropathy
Juvenile chronic arthritis
Erosive osteoarthritis
- Crystal deposition arthropathy
Hydroxyapatite joint disease (m.c.)
Calcium pyrophosphate dihydrate crystal deposition
disease
Hemochromatosis
Gout
- Degenerative joint disease
Secondary osteoarthritis (m.c.)
Primary osteoarthritis
Diffuse idiopathic skeletal hyperostosis
Ossification of the posterior longitudinal ligament

- Neuropathic arthropathy
- Connective tissue arthropathies
    Systemic lupus erythematosus
    Progressive systemic sclerosis
    Mixed connective tissue disease
- Miscellaneous
    Fibromyalgia syndrome
    Pigmented villonodular synovitis
    Synovial chondrometaplasia
    Hemophilic arthropathy
- Infection
    Suppurative
    Tuberculous

5.11 Arthritides Affecting the Spine

Arthritis	Joints Commonly Affected
Degenerative joint disease	Entire spine
Ankylosing spondylitis	Entire spine
Reiter's syndrome	Thoracolumbar, sacroiliac
Juvenile chronic arthritis	Cervical
Rheumatoid arthritis	Cervical
Arthritis associated with psoriasis	Thoracolumbar, sacroiliac
Arthritis asscoiated with enteropathy	Thoracolumbar, sacroiliac
Diffuse idiopathic skeletal hyperostosis	Cervicothoracic
Infectious spondylitis	Thoracolumbar
Neuropathic arthropathy	Lumbar

5.12 Arthritides Commonly Affecting the Hands

Arthritis	Joints Commonly Affected
Rheumatoid arthritis	Metacarpophalangeal, proximal interphalangeal joints
Arthritis associated with psoriasis	Distal interphalangeal joints
Erosive osteoarthritis	Distal interphalangeal, proximal interphalangeal, first metacarpophalangeal joints
Calcium pyrophosphate crystal deposition disease	Metacarpophalangeal joints
Systemic lupus erythematosus	Metacarpophalangeal, proximal interphalangeal joints
Progressive systemic sclerosis	Metacarpophalangeal joints

5.13 Arthritides Commonly Affecting the Feet

Arthritis	Joints Commonly Affected
Rheumatoid arthritis	Metatarsophalangeal, proximal interphalangeal joints
Reiter's syndrome	Metatarsophalangeal, proximal interphalangeal joints
Gouty arthritis	First metatarsophalangeal joint
Degenerative joint disease	First metatarsophalangeal joint
Neuropathic arthropathy	Midfoot

5.14 Diseases Affecting the Sacroiliac Joints

- Bilateral
    Degenerative joint disease (m.c.)
    Ankylosing spondylitis (symmetric)
    Reiter's syndrome (asymmetric)

Arthritis associated with psoriasis (asymmetric)
Arthritis associated with enteropathy (asymmetric)
Hyperparathyroidism (symmetric)
Osteitis condensans ilii
- Unilateral
Infectious arthritis
Gouty arthritis
Rheumatoid arthritis

5.15 Diseases Affecting the Atlantoaxial Articulation

- Trauma (m.c.)
- Arthritides
Rheumatoid arthritis
Ankylosing spondylitis
Reiter's syndrome
Arthritis associated with psoriasis
Arthritis associated with enteropathy
Juvenile chronic arthritis
- Congenital
Isolated agenesis of the transverse ligament
Trisomy 21 with agenesis of the transverse ligament
Atlanto-occipital assimilation
Odontoid hypoplasia
Os odontoideum
Os terminale
- Infection
Retropharyngeal abscess
- Miscellaneous
Grisel's syndrome

5.16 Signs of Unstable Spinal Lesions

Subluxation of greater than 3 mm or 25%
Sagittal rotation of greater than 11 degrees
Vertebral body compression greater than 25%
Atlantodental interspace greater than 3 mm (adults)/
   greater than 5 mm (children younger than 14 years)
Retropulsion of bone fragments into the spinal canal

5.17 Unstable Spinal Lesions

- Cervical spine
    Type II/III odontoid fracture (Type II m.c.)
    Os odontoideum
    Flexion teardrop fracture
    Extension teardrop fracture (in extension)
    Burst fracture
    Bilateral facet dislocation
- Thoracolumbar spine
    Burst fracture
    Bilateral facet dislocation
    Chance fracture

5.18 Congenital Anomalies of the Spine

- Cervical
    Atlanto-occipital assimilation
    Block vertebra
    Cervical rib
    Klippel-Feil syndrome

  Os terminale
  Os odontoideum
  Posterior ponticle
  Spina bifida
- Thoracic
  Block vertebra
  Spina bifida
  Diastematomyelia
  Butterfly vertebra
  Hemivertebra
- Lumbar
  Asymmetric facet plane orientation
  Lumbosacral transitional segment
  Spina bifida
  Block vertebra

5.19 Causes of Avascular Necrosis of Bone

Trauma
Chronic steroid therapy/Cushing's syndrome
Alcoholism
Pancreatitis
Sickle cell anemia
Systemic lupus erythematosus
Caisson disease
Radiation therapy

5.20 Common Locations for Avascular Necrosis of Bone

Joint	Location within Joint
Knee	Medial femoral condyle
Ankle	Dome of the talus
Foot	Navicular, second metatarsal head
Wrist	Lunate, scaphoid
Elbow	Capitulum
Hip	Femoral head
Shoulder	Humeral head

5.21 Radiation Exposure from Common Diagnostic Procedures

Procedure	Estimated Whole-Body Dosage (mrem)
Chest	10
Skull	40
Cervical spine	50
Lumbar spine	130
Thoracic spine	240
Mammogram	450

Part III

Selected Disorders

Chapter 6

Selected Neurologic Disorders

6.1 Acoustic Neuroma

Benign tumor of cranial nerve VIII

Epidemiology/Etiology

30 to 50-year age group
Associated with neurofibromatosis

Signs/Symptoms

Hearing loss
Vertigo
Ipsilateral cranial nerve V and VII lesions

Diagnosis

Magnetic resonance imaging

6.2 Acquired Immunodeficiency Syndrome (AIDS)

Infection with the human immunodeficiency virus (HIV), which leads to multiorgan manifestations and almost always death. Neurologic manifestations may occur in up to two-thirds of cases.

Epidemiology/Etiology

Usually younger than 60 years old
Males more than females
High-risk groups
> Homosexual/bisexual men
> Bisexual women
> Transfusion recipients
> Intravenous drug abusers
> Persons with multiple sex partners

Signs/Symptoms

Opportunistic infections
> Viral (cytomegalovirus, herpes simplex, varicella zoster)
> Nonviral (*Candida, Toxoplasmosis, Mycobacterium, Histoplasma, Aspergillus, Pneumocystis carinii pneumonia*)

Neoplasms
> Primary central nervous system lymphoma
> Metastatic lymphoma
> Metastatic Kaposi's sarcoma

Meningitis
Encephalitis
Myelopathy
Peripheral neuropathy
Cerebral infarction and hemorrhage
AIDS dementia

Diagnosis

Serum HIV testing

6.3 Alzheimer's Disease

A chronic form of presenile dementia of unknown etiology with severe neuropsychologic manifestations and eventually death

Epidemiology/Etiology

Fifth decade
Females more than males
Lasts 2 to 5 years

Signs/Symptoms

Memory disturbance
Disorientation
Confusion
Dementia
Anxiety
Hallucinations
Agitation

Diagnosis

Negative complete blood count, serum chemistry
Normal vitamin B-12 and folic acid levels
Normal thyroid function studies
Normal lumbar puncture
Electroencephalogram
+/– Cerebral atrophy on computed tomography/magnetic
  resonance imaging

6.4 Amyotrophic Lateral Sclerosis (ALS)

A neurologic disorder of unknown etiology in which the manifestations are those of a combination of muscular atrophy with spastic paraplegia. Spinal findings usually occur first, consistently followed by bulbar palsy. Damage occurs in the anterior horn cells, bulbar motor nuclei, and pyramidal and corticobulbar tracts.

Epidemiology/Etiology

40 to 65 years old
Males more than females

Signs/Symptoms

Muscular atrophy
Fasciculations (characteristic feature)
Bulbar palsy
    Palsy of cranial nerves IX, X, XI, XII
Dysphagia (neurogenic)
Dysphasia
Spasticity (may be mild)
Pyramidal tract signs
Rapidly progressive and fatal (75 to 85% die within 3 years)

Diagnosis

Electromyography
Elevated creatine phosphokinase levels
Normal cerebrospinal fluid
Abnormal glucose tolerance/glucose loading tests

6.5 Aneurysm

Abnormal dilation of an intracranial blood vessel (Figure 6-1)

Epidemiology/Etiology

Any age group depending on etiology
Congenital ("berry" aneurysm)
Atherosclerosis
Traumatic
Mycotic
Neoplasm

Signs/Symptoms

Cranial nerve palsies (especially cranial nerve III)
Headache
Seizures
Signs/symptoms of subarachnoid hemorrhage if ruptured

Diagnosis

Magnetic resonance imaging
Angiography
Computed tomography

6.6 Arnold-Chiari Malformation

Malformation consisting of caudal displacement of the brainstem and a portion of the cerebellum through the foramen magnum into the cervical spinal canal

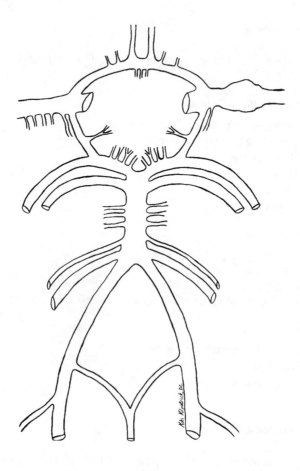

Figure 6-1 Aneurysm of the Right Middle Cerebral Artery (Note: Circle of Willis seen from above). *Source:* Copyright © 1993 by Kiki Kilpatrick, D.C.

Epidemiology/Etiology

Congenital

Signs/Symptoms

Usually asymptomatic until adulthood
Low cranial nerve palsies
Upper motor neuron lesion findings
Often associated with spina bifida and hydrocephalus

Diagnosis

Magnetic resonance imaging
Computed tomography

6.7 Arteriovenous Malformation

Abnormal conglomeration of wide feeding and draining blood vessels often separated by a mesh of capillaries, often with arteriovenous shunts

Epidemiology/Etiology

Congenital
Symptoms usually begin in 10 to 30-year age group

Signs/Symptoms

May be asymptomatic
Subarachnoid hemorrhage
Seizures
Headache
Murmur synchronous with pulse auscultated over orbits
Linear calcification on skull radiographs (15 to 30%)

Diagnosis

Magnetic resonance imaging
Computed tomography
Angiography is definitive

6.8 Astrocytomas

Most common form of brain tumor

Epidemiology/Etiology

30 to 60-year age group
Graded I to IV
Grade IV is a glioblastoma multiforme (highly malignant)

Signs/Symptoms

Seizures
Headaches (diffuse, nocturnal)
Papilledema
Behavioral changes

Diagnosis

Magnetic resonance imaging
Computed tomography
Biopsy

6.9 Basilar Invagination

Cephalization of the odontoid process through the
foramen magnum

Epidemiology/Etiology

Congenital
Osteomalacia
Inflammatory arthropathies (e.g., rheumatoid arthritis)
Paget's disease of bone

Signs/Symptoms

Many are asymptomatic
Slowly progressive
Lower cranial nerve palsies
Upper motor neuron lesion signs/symptoms
May mimic multiple sclerosis

Diagnosis

Violation of Chamberlain's/Macgregor's lines on plain film
    radiography
Magnetic resonance imaging
Computed tomography

6.10 Benign Intracranial Hypertension

Papilledema without a known cause; also known as
pseudotumor cerebri

Epidemiology/Etiology

Female more than male
Obese women

Signs/Symptoms

   Papilledema
   Headache
   Nausea/vomiting
   Giddiness
   Enlarged blind spot

Diagnosis

   Magnetic resonance imaging (normal)
   Computed tomography (normal)

6.11 Cerebrovascular Accident

   Permanent brain damage secondary to ischemia or
   hemorrhage; also known as a stroke

Epidemiology/Etiology

   70 to 80-year age group
   Males same as females
   Thromboembolic disease
   Hypertension

Signs/Symptoms

   Acute onset
   Hemiplegia
   Slurred speech
   Unconsciousness (50%)
   Headache
   Seizure (20%)

Facial paralysis
Nausea/vomiting

Diagnosis

Magnetic resonance imaging
Computed tomography

6.12 Cluster Headache

Hemicranial headaches that occur in clusters during
certain specific periods of time or seasons; also known as a
histamine headache

Epidemiology/Etiology

Men more than women
Family history in 20%

Signs/Symptoms

Very sudden onset
Severe unilateral pain
Usually supraorbital region
Usually experience one to three attacks in 1 day
Last 1 to 2 hours
Redness of the ipsilateral eye
Ipsilateral lacrimation
Ipsilateral rhinorrhea
Photophobia

Diagnosis

Clinical presentation is classic

6.13 Concussion

Traumatic impact of the brain with the skull

Epidemiology/Etiology

Trauma

Signs/Symptoms

Altered level of consciousness
Amnesia, usually retrograde
Vomiting
Transient loss of complete mental function

Diagnosis

Magnetic resonance imaging to rule out cerebral damage

6.14 Craniopharyngioma

Benign suprasellar tumor of the remnants of Rathke's pouch

Epidemiology/Etiology

5 to 20-year age group
Tumor of the remnants of Rathke's pouch

Signs/Symptoms

Endocrine disturbances
Bitemporal hemianopia
Optic nerve atrophy
Hydrocephalus

Behavioral disturbances
Diabetes insipidus

Diagnosis

Computed tomography (tumor commonly calcifies)

6.15 Encephalitis

Inflammation of the brain

Epidemiology/Etiology

Infectious (e.g., viral)

Signs/Symptoms

Fever
Headache
Nuchal rigidity
Altered level of consciousness
Photophobia
Vomiting
Seizures

Diagnosis

Lumbar puncture with culture and sensitivity
Electroencephalogram
Complete blood count

6.16 Ependymoma

Benign tumor of ependymal cells

Epidemiology/Etiology

   Children and young adults
   Fourth ventricle (often inoperable)
   Lumbar spinal cord

Signs/Symptoms

   Brain
      Hydrocephalus
      Ataxia
      Dysdiadochokinesia
      Other cerebellar signs
   Spinal cord
      Conus medullaris syndrome

Diagnosis

   Magnetic resonance imaging
   Biopsy

6.17 Epilepsy

   Abnormal cerebral neuron function resulting in attacks of
   disturbance of consciousness and altered motor activity

Epidemiology/Etiology

   Idiopathic (m.c.)
   Trauma
   Ischemia
   Space-occupying intracranial lesions
   Inflammation

Signs/Symptoms

   Vary with type of seizure
   Some have premonitory symptoms
   Tonic/clonic movements
   Disturbed consciousness with motor symptoms

Diagnosis

   Electroencephalogram
   Magnetic resonance imaging to rule out intracranial disease

6.18 Guillain-Barré Syndrome

   Acute idiopathic polyneuropathy

Epidemiology/Etiology

   Any age group
   Idiopathic

Signs/Symptoms

   Commonly preceded by upper respiratory infection
   Multifocal paresthesias
   Ascending flaccid paralysis
   Hyporeflexia
   Muscle atrophy
   May cause cranial nerve palsies
   Painful

Diagnosis

   Clinical findings are typical

6.19 Medulloblastoma

Malignant childhood cerebellar tumor

Epidemiology/Etiology

Childhood, adolescence

Signs/Symptoms

Ataxia
Poor balance
Nystagmus
Signs and symptoms of increased intracranial pressure

Diagnosis

Magnetic resonance imaging

6.20 Meniere's Disease

Syndrome of vertigo, tinnitus, and deafness

Epidemiology/Etiology

20 to 50-year age group
Male same as female

Signs/Symptoms

Paroxysmal onset
Vertigo
Tinnitus
Sensorineural deafness
Nausea and vomiting
Nystagmus

Diagnosis

Clinical findings are typical
Magnetic resonance imaging to rule out cranial nerve VIII
disease

6.21 Meningioma

Benign tumor of the meninges

Epidemiology/Etiology

40 to 60-year age group
Female more than male

Signs/Symptoms

Dependent on site
Seizures
Headache
Nausea and vomiting

Diagnosis

Computed tomography (tumor commonly calcifies)

6.22 Meningitis

Infection of the meninges of the brain and/or spinal cord,
usually with a rapid course

Epidemiology/Etiology

Any age group

Bacteria
Aseptic (acute form caused by a virus)

Signs/Symptoms

Fever
Nuchal rigidity
Headache
Altered mental status
Vomiting
Photophobia
Often after a recent respiratory tract infection

Diagnosis

Lumbar puncture with culture and sensitivity
Complete blood count
Blood culture

6.23 Migraine Headache

Group of vasomotor headaches characterized by repeated attacks

Epidemiology/Etiology

Women more than men
Vasoconstriction followed by vasodilation of intracranial arteries

Signs/Symptoms

Dependent on type
Unilateral throbbing headache

Premonitory symptoms common (auditory, visual, smell)
Nausea/vomiting
Photophobia

Diagnosis

Symptom complex is typical
Magnetic resonance imaging to rule out intracranial disease

6.24 Multiple Sclerosis

A progressive and usually fatal multifocal demyelinating central nervous system disease characterized by plaque formation

Epidemiology/Etiology

Most common demyelinating disease
10 to 50-year age group
Female to male 2:1

Signs/Symptoms

Exacerbations and remissions
Upper motor neuron lesion findings
Spasticity
Sensory disturbances
Optic neuritis
Vertigo
Ataxia
Bowel and bladder dysfunction
Cranial nerve palsies
Seizures

Impotence
Hearing loss

Diagnosis

Magnetic resonance imaging
Lumbar puncture (increased gamma globulin, lymphocytes,
and protein)

6.25 Myasthenia Gravis

Membrane disturbance of the motor endplate, resulting
in classic clinical picture

Epidemiology/Etiology

20 to 40-year age group
Female more than male

Signs/Symptoms

Increasing muscle fatigue/paresis/paralysis with exercise
Recovery with rest
Ocular, soft palate, and throat muscles commonly involved
early

Diagnosis

Immediate resolution with cholinesterase inhibitor injection
Mediastinal computed tomography to rule out thymoma in
adults

6.26 Parkinson's Disease

A progressive, usually fatal central nervous system disease characterized by tremors and akinesia

Epidemiology/Etiology

Males more than females
Onset in fifth decade
Degeneration of substantia nigra
Familial
Postencephalopathy
Arteriosclerosis
Drug-induced
Idiopathic

Signs/Symptoms

Festinating gait
Cogwheel rigidity
"Stooped over" posture
Resting tremor (especially "pill rolling" tremor)
Disturbed affectivity
Speech disturbances

Diagnosis

Patient presentation is classic

6.27 Pernicious Anemia

Vitamin B-12 deficiency resulting in classic neuropathy called subacute combined degeneration of the spinal cord

Epidemiology/Etiology

Alcoholism
Gastrointestinal disease

Signs/Symptoms

Abnormal proprioception and vibration sense
Painful lower extremity paresthesia
Ataxia
Upper motor neuron lesion signs
Megaloblastic anemia

Diagnosis

Serum vitamin B-12 level
Complete blood count

6.28 Pituitary Adenoma

Benign tumor of the pituitary gland

Epidemiology/Etiology

30 to 50-year age group
Eosinophilic, basophilic, chromophobe types

Signs/Symptoms

Acromegaly with eosinophilic adenoma
Endocrine disturbances
Sellar enlargement
Bitemporal hemianopia

Diagnosis

Magnetic resonance imaging

6.29 Spinal Canal Stenosis

Narrowing of the spinal canal

Epidemiology/Etiology

Congenital
Degenerative joint disease

Signs/Symptoms

Symptoms may occur only with extension of the spine
Muscular weakness in multilevel distribution
Sensory disturbances in multilevel distribution
Upper motor neuron lesion signs

Diagnosis

Computed tomography
Magnetic resonance imaging

6.30 Subarachnoid Hemorrhage

Bleeding into the subarachnoid space

Epidemiology/Etiology

55 to 60-year age group
Intracranial aneurysm (m.c.)
Trauma

Ruptured arteriovenous malformation
Neoplasms

Signs/Symptoms

Sudden severe headache
Altered level of consciousness
Meningeal signs
Seizures
Papilledema

Diagnosis

Computed tomography
Magnetic resonance imaging
Angiography
Lumbar puncture if computed tomography/magnetic
resonance imaging are negative

6.31 Subluxation

An alteration of the normal biodynamics of a joint,
resulting in dyskinesia and its sequelae

Epidemiology/Etiology

Any age group
Trauma
Congenital
Arthritides
Scoliosis
Muscle spasm
Sprain/strain

Signs/Symptoms

   Pain
   Paresthesia
   Reflex muscle spasm
   Decreased range of motion
   Visceral effects (controversial)

Diagnosis

   Clinical presentation is classic
   Plain film radiography to rule out aggressive pathology

6.32 Syringomyelia

   Cystic dilation of the central canal of the spinal cord

Epidemiology/Etiology

   Associated with
      Trauma
      Congenital spinal cord anomalies

Signs/Symptoms

   Dependent on spinal region affected
   Loss of pain and temperature
   Spastic paresis/paralysis
   Dissociation of sensation
   Neuropathic joints

Diagnosis

   Magnetic resonance imaging

6.33 Transient Ischemic Attacks

Transient neurologic deficits secondary to ischemia with no permanent neurologic damage

Epidemiology/Etiology

Atherosclerosis (m.c.)
Age older than 40 years

Signs/Symptoms

Syncope
Amaurosis fugax
Paresthesia
Weakness
Aphasia

Diagnosis

Carotid Doppler ultrasound
Magnetic resonance imaging (normal)

Chapter 7

Selected Skeletal Disorders

7.1 Acromegaly (Figure 7-1)

The production of excess growth hormone by a pituitary adenoma after the cessation of skeletal growth with resultant effects on the skeleton

Category

Nutritional, metabolic, endocrine

General

Osseous enlargement
Soft tissue enlargement
Osteopenia
Precocious degenerative joint disease
Enthesopathy

Laboratory

Elevated plasma growth hormone levels
Abnormal glucose tolerance

Hands

"Spade-like" hands

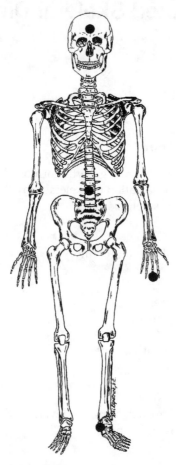

Figure 7-1 Skeletal Distribution of Changes Associated with Acromegaly. *Source:* Copyright © 1993 by Kiki Kilpatrick, D.C.

Enlarged terminal tufts
Cystic changes in carpal bones

Spine

Posterior vertebral body scalloping

Skull

Enlarged sella turcica
Overpneumatization of paranasal sinuses
Enlarged external occipital protuberance
Prognathism
Thickened cranial vault

Foot

Increased heel pad thickness (>23 mm)

7.2 Aneurysmal Bone Cyst (Figures 7-2 and 7-3)

Tumor-like cystic dilation of bone that some believe to be post-traumatic in etiology; has the appearance of an aneurysm, therefore its namesake

Category

Tumor/tumor-like (benign)

General

May arise within a pre-existing lesion
Not a true tumor
Painful scoliosis
Only known benign bone tumor that extends from one bone to another

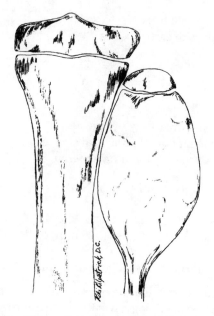

Figure 7-2 Aneurysmal Bone Cyst of the Proximal Fibula. *Source:* Copyright © 1993 by Kiki Kilpatrick, D.C.

Epidemiology

    10 to 30 years old; peaks at age 16 years
    Female to male 1.5:1

Location

    Tibia
    Femur

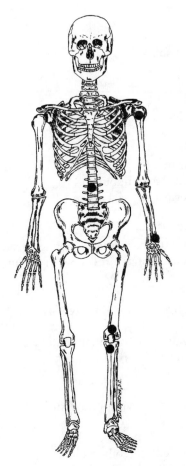

Figure 7-3 Skeletal Distribution of Aneurysmal Bone Cyst. *Source:* Copyright ©
1993 by Kiki Kilpatrick, D.C.

Humerus
Radius
Neural arch of spine

Radiographic Features

Metaphyseal
Eccentrically located
Purely lytic
Highly expansile
Thin cortical rim
Multiloculated ("soap bubble")
Usually no periosteal reaction

Differential Diagnosis

Giant cell tumor (subarticular, older age group)
Simple bone cyst (nonpainful, slow-growing)

7.3 Ankylosing Spondylitis (Figure 7-4)

Idiopathic autoimmune inflammatory arthropathy that particularly affects the axial skeleton

Category

Arthritides (seronegative spondyloarthropathy)

General

Usually begins with sacroiliac joints
Atlantoaxial instability is possible
Bilaterally symmetric disease

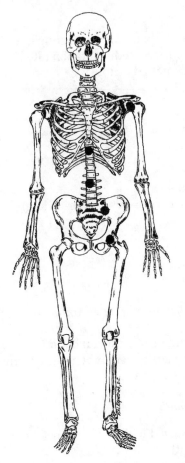

Figure 7-4 Skeletal Distribution of Ankylosing Spondylitis. *Source:* Copyright © 1993 by Kiki Kilpatrick, D.C.

Laboratory

Positive histocompatibility locus antigen-B27 (90%)
Elevated erythrocyte sedimentation rate
Negative rheumatoid factor

Epidemiology

Young males

Location

Sacroiliac joints
Thoracolumbar spine (cervical spine late)
Hips
Shoulders

Radiographic Features

Sacroiliitis
Thin vertical syndesmophyte production
Bony fusion
Erosions at corners of vertebral bodies (Romanus lesion)
Sclerosis at corners of vertebral bodies (shiny corner sign)
Periarticular osteopenia

Differential Diagnosis

Arthritis associated with psoriasis (asymmetric, acral involvement)
Reiter's syndrome (asymmetric, lower extremity predominates, clinical triad)

7.4 Arthritis Associated with Enteropathy (Figure 7-5)

Inflammatory spinal arthropathy associated with inflammatory bowel disease

Category

Arthritides (seronegative spondyloarthropathy)

General

Associated with ulcerative colitis, Crohn's disease, and
   irritable bowel syndrome
Atlantoaxial instability is possible

Laboratory

Positive histocompatibility locus antigen-B27
Elevated erythrocyte sedimentation rate
Negative rheumatoid factor
Abnormal laboratory tests associated with enteropathy

Epidemiology

15 to 50-year age group

Location

Sacroiliac joints
Spine
Lower extremity joints

Radiographic Features

Bilateral but asymmetric sacroiliitis
Thick parasyndesmophytes

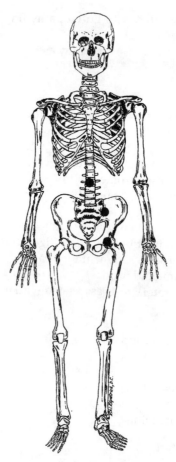

Figure 7-5 Skeletal Distribution of Arthritis Associated with Enteropathy.
Source: Copyright © 1993 by Kiki Kilpatrick, D.C.

Osseous fusion
Bony erosions

Differential Diagnosis

Ankylosing spondylitis (thin vertical syndesmophytes)
Reiter's syndrome (classic clinical triad)
Arthritis associated with psoriasis (psoriasis, nail changes)

7.5 Arthritis Associated with Psoriasis (Figure 7-6)

An idiopathic autoimmune inflammatory arthropathy
associated with psoriasis

Category

Arthritides (seronegative spondyloarthropathy)

General

Associated with nail pitting
Bilateral but asymmetric disease
Atlantoaxial instability is possible

Laboratory

Positive histocompatibility locus antigen-B27
Elevated erythrocyte sedimentation rate
Negative rheumatoid factor

Epidemiology

15% of patients with psoriasis develop this arthritis
Males and females affected
30 to 50-year age group

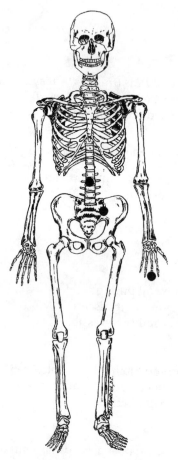

Figure 7-6 Skeletal Distribution of Arthritis Associated with Psoriasis. *Source:* Copyright © 1993 by Kiki Kilpatrick, D.C.

Location

Hands (distal interphalangeal joints)
Sacroiliac joints
Spine

Radiographic Features

Sacroiliitis
Thick parasyndesmophytes
Osseous fusion
Joint erosions
Terminal phalangeal sclerosis
Periosteal reaction

Differential Diagnosis

Ankylosing spondylitis (symmetry, primarily axial, thin
vertical syndesmophytes)
Reiter's syndrome (lower extremity predominates, clinical
triad)

7.6 Battered Child Syndrome (Figure 7-7)

Child abuse

Category

Trauma

General

Multiple injuries at different stages of healing

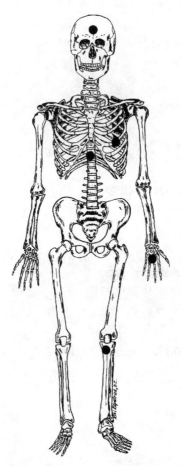

Figure 7-7 Skeletal Distribution of Battered Child Syndrome. *Source:* Copyright © 1993 by Kiki Kilpatrick, D.C.

Epidemiology

20% have skeletal trauma

Location

Thorax
Skull
Spine
Tibia
Metacarpals

Radiographic Features

Multiple fractures at different stages of healing
Metaphyseal/epiphyseal fractures
"Corner" fractures
Rib fractures
Skull fractures
Avulsion fractures
Subdural hematoma

Differential Diagnosis

Accidental injury (usually singular, same stage of healing if
multiple)

7.7 Calcium Pyrophosphate Crystal Deposition Disease (Figure 7-8)

Deposition of calcium pyrophosphate dihydrate crystals
in joints with resultant inflammatory arthropathy

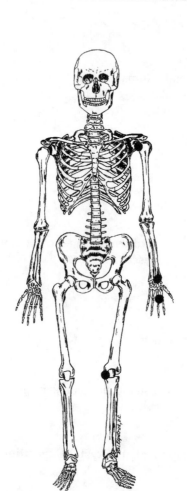

Figure 7-8 Skeletal Distribution of Calcium Pyrophosphate Crystal Deposition Disease. *Source:* Copyright © 1993 by Kiki Kilpatrick, D.C.

Category

Arthritides (crystal deposition arthropathy)

General

Associated with hyperparathyroidism, hemochromatosis, gout

Degenerative joint disease in a joint that does not normally develop the disease

Joint aspiration is definitive

Laboratory

Abnormalities associated with primary disease (e.g., hyperparathyroidism)

Epidemiology

Adults

Males and females

Location

Knee

Wrist

Metacarpophalangeal joints

Shoulder

Radiographic Features

Chondrocalcinosis

Degenerative joint disease

Periarticular calcifications (ligaments, tendons, synovium, capsule)

Differential Diagnosis

> Neuropathic arthropathy (underlying disease, more severe changes)
> Degenerative joint disease (weight-bearing joints)
> Gout (tophi)

7.8 Chondroblastoma (Figures 7-9 and 7-10)

Childhood tumor composed of chondroblasts

Category

> Tumor/tumor-like (benign)

General

> One of only a few epiphyseal lesions
> Can cross the physis
> Painful

Epidemiology

> 5 to 25-year age group
> Male to female 2:1

Location

> Femur
> Tibia
> Humerus

Radiographic Features

> Ovoid geographic lucency

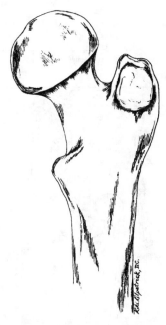

Figure 7-9 Chondroblastoma of the Greater Trochanter of the Femur. *Source:*
Copyright © 1993 by Kiki Kilpatrick, D.C.

Sclerotic margin
Calcification (25 to 50%)
Epiphyseal/apophyseal

Differential Diagnosis

Giant cell tumor (older age group)
Fungal infection (history, fever)

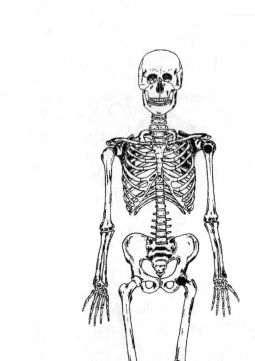

Figure 7-10 Skeletal Distribution of Chondroblastoma. *Source:* Copyright © 1993 by Kiki Kilpatrick, D.C.

7.9 Chondromyxoid Fibroma

Rare tumor of chondroid, fibroid, and myxoid tissue

Category

Tumor/tumor-like (benign)

General

Slowly progressive
Painful
May cross physis

Epidemiology

10 to 30-year age group
Male to female 1:1

Location

Tibia
Femur
Pelvis
Short tubular bones

Radiographic Features

Metaphyseal
Slowly expansile
Ovoid lucency
Eccentrically located
Long axis parallel to long axis of host bone
Eccentric thick sclerotic border
Calcification (late)
No periosteal reaction

Differential Diagnosis

Aneurysmal bone cyst (thin cortex, rapidly expansile)
Solitary bone cyst (centrally located, painless unless fractured)
Fibroxanthoma (painless, more scalloped inner margin)
Fibrous dysplasia (painless)

7.10 Chondrosarcoma (Figure 7-11)

Primary malignant skeletal neoplasm of chondroid origin

Category

Tumor/tumor-like (malignant)

General

Third most common primary skeletal malignancy
May arise *de novo* or within a benign lesion
Painful

Epidemiology

30 to 60-year age group
Male to female 2:1

Location

Pelvis
Femur
Scapula
Ribs
Humerus

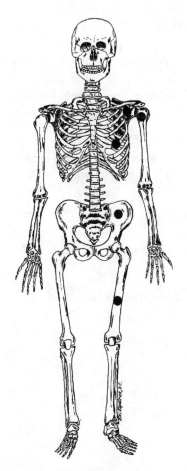

Figure 7-11 Skeletal Distribution of Chondrosarcoma. *Source:* Copyright ©
1993 by Kiki Kilpatrick, D.C.

Radiographic Features

   Metaphyseal/diaphyseal
   Expansile lucency with cortical destruction
   Sclerotic margin
   Internal calcification (two-thirds of cases)
   Soft tissue mass; usually large

Differential Diagnosis

   Osteochondroma (contiguous with cortex)
   Enchondroma (no soft tissue mass)

7.11 Chordoma (Figure 7-12)

   Malignant neoplasm of the remnants of the notochord

Category

   Tumor/tumor-like (malignant)

General

   Headache
   Sacral pain

Epidemiology

   40 to 60-year age group

Location

   Sacrum
   Clivus
   Vertebra

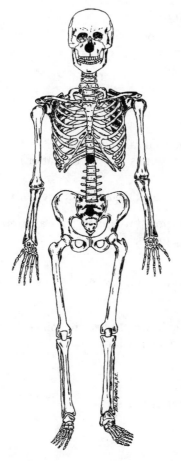

Figure 7-12 Skeletal Distribution of Chordoma. *Source:* Copyright © 1993 by
Kiki Kilpatrick, D.C.

Radiographic Features

    Expansile lytic lesion
    Multiloculated
    Scalloped margins
    Calcification
    Soft tissue mass

Differential Diagnosis

    Giant cell tumor (no calcification)
    Metastasis (nonexpansile, no calcification)

7.12 Degenerative Joint Disease (Figure 7-13)

    Noninflammatory "wear and tear" arthropathy of weight-bearing joints.

Category

    Arthritides (noninflammatory)

General

    Typically found in weight-bearing joints
    Primary and secondary forms

Epidemiology

    Age older than 40 years
    Males more than females

Location

    Spine
    Hips
    Knees

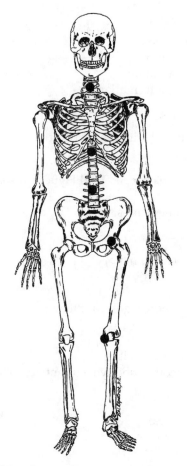

Figure 7-13 Skeletal Distribution of Degenerative Joint Disease. *Source:* Copyright © 1993 by Kiki Kilpatrick, D.C.

Radiographic Features

Eccentric loss of joint space
Subarticular sclerosis
Osteophyte formation
Subarticular cyst formation

Differential Diagnosis

Commonly found with other arthritides

7.13 Diffuse Idiopathic Skeletal Hyperostosis (Figure 7-14)

Ossifying diathesis most commonly affecting the spine

Category

Arthritis (noninflammatory)

General

Joint stiffness more significant than pain

Laboratory

25% have diabetes mellitus
Positive histocompatibility locus antigen-B27 in one-third

Epidemiology

Older than 50 years of age
Males more than females

Location

Thoracic spine

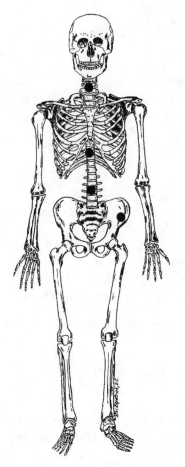

Figure 7-14 Skeletal Distribution of Diffuse Idiopathic Skeletal Hyperostosis.
Source: Copyright © 1993 by Kiki Kilpatrick, D.C.

Cervical spine
Pelvis
Lumbar spine

Radiographic Features

Diffuse flowing anterolateral vertebral hyperostosis
Preservation of facet joints and disc spaces
Enthesopathy
Bridging of symphysis pubis

Differential Diagnosis

Fluorosis (skeletal opacification)
Ankylosing spondylitis (facet joint involvement, thin
vertical syndesmophytes)
Degenerative joint disease (posterior joint involvement, disc
space narrowing)

7.14 Enchondroma (Figures 7-15 and 7-16)

Benign medullary skeletal neoplasm of chondroid origin

Category

Tumor/tumor-like (benign)

General

Most common tumor of the bones of the hand
Associated with soft tissue hemangiomas (Maffucci's
syndrome)
Hereditary polyostotic form (enchondromatosis [Ollier's
disease])

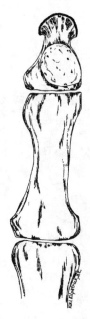

Figure 7-15 Enchondroma of a Phalanx. *Source:* Copyright © 1993 by Kiki Kilpatrick, D.C.

Epidemiology

    10 to 30-year age group
    Males same as females

Location

    Hands
    Femur

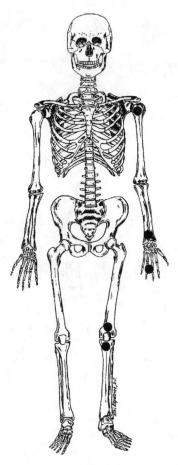

Figure 7-16 Skeletal Distribution of Enchondroma. *Source:* Copyright © 1993 by Kiki Kilpatrick, D.C.

Humerus
Tibia
Radius
Ulna

Radiographic Features

Metaphyseal/diaphyseal
Geographic ovoid lucency
Central calcification ("rings and broken rings")
Endosteal scalloping
May be expansile

Differential Diagnosis

Solitary bone cyst (rare in hands)
Bone infarction (differentiation difficult in long bones)
Chondrosarcoma (differentiation difficult in long bones)

7.15 Eosinophilic Granuloma (Figure 7-17)

Deposition of eosinophils, histiocytes, and reticulum cells, primarily in bone

Category

Tumor/tumor-like (benign)

General

Form of histiocytosis X
Localized to bone
Usually solitary
Spontaneous resolution in 12 to 18 months

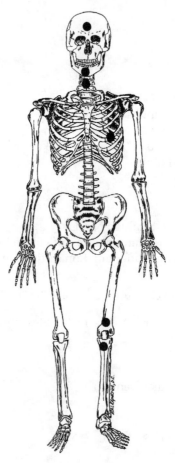

Figure 7-17 Skeletal Distribution of Eosinophilic Granuloma. *Source:* Copyright © 1993 by Kiki Kilpatrick, D.C.

Epidemiology

 5 to 10-year age group
 Male to female 1.5:1

Location

 Skull (m.c.)
 Spine
 Mandible
 Ribs
 Femur
 Tibia

Radiographic Features

 Geographic lucency
 +/– Thin sclerotic rim
 Beveled edges
 Button sequestrum (skull)
 Collapsed vertebra

7.16 Ewing's Sarcoma (Figure 7-18)

 Primary malignant round cell skeletal tumor of children

Category

 Tumor/tumor-like (malignant)

General

 Clinically and radiographically mimics osteomyelitis

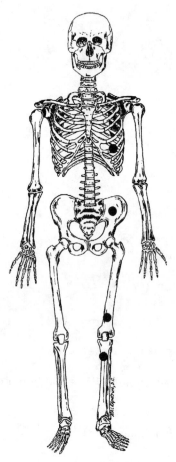

Figure 7-18 Skeletal Distribution of Ewing's Sarcoma. *Source:* Copyright ©
1993 by Kiki Kilpatrick, D.C.

Laboratory

Elevated white blood cell count

Epidemiology

5 to 15-year age group
Male to female 1.5:1

Location

Humerus
Femur
Pelvis
Ribs

Radiographic Features

Metaphyseal/diaphyseal
Moth-eaten/permeative bone destruction
Laminated periosteal reaction
Soft tissue mass
+/– New bone formation

Differential Diagnosis

Osteomyelitis (differentiation difficult)
Neuroblastoma (age younger than 5 years)
Osteosarcoma (older age group, opacification)

7.17 Fibrosarcoma (Figure 7-19)

Primary malignant skeletal neoplasm of fibrous tissue origin

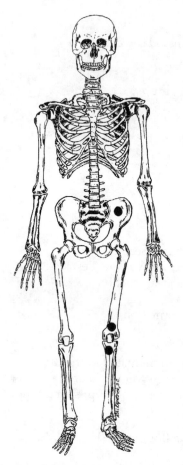

Figure 7-19 Skeletal Distribution of Fibrosarcoma. *Source:* Copyright © 1993 by Kiki Kilpatrick, D.C.

Category

Tumor/tumor-like (malignant)

General

May arise *de novo* or in a benign lesion

Epidemiology

30 to 60-year age group
Male to female 1:1

Location

Femur
Tibia
Pelvis

Radiographic Features

Geographic to permeative lucency
Thinned expanded cortex
Soft tissue mass

Differential Diagnosis

Malignant fibrous histiocytoma (differentiation difficult)
Multiple myeloma (usually diffuse)
Lymphoma (blastic)
Metastasis (differentiation difficult)

7.18 Fibrous Dysplasia (Figure 7-20)

Idiopathic developmental fibrous replacement of bone

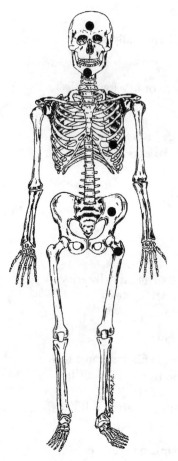

Figure 7-20 Skeletal Distribution of Fibrous Dysplasia. *Source:* Copyright © 1993 by Kiki Kilpatrick, D.C.

Category

Unknown

General

Great imitator of other bone diseases
Polyostotic form with precocious puberty (McCune-Albright syndrome)
Most common cause of expansile rib lesion

Epidemiology

5 to 15-year age group
Male same as female

Location

Femur
Pelvis
Ribs
Skull
Mandible

Radiographic Features

Metaphyseal
Geographic "ground glass" lucency
Thick sclerotic rim
Sclerotic in skull base/mandible (cherubism)
Coxa vara (Sheppard's crook deformity)

Differential Diagnosis

Most known bone lesions

7.19 Fibroxanthoma (Figure 7-21)

Abnormal deposition of fibrous tissue in cortical bone

Category

Tumor/tumor-like (benign)

General

Two types: fibrous cortical defect, nonossifying fibroma
Common childhood tumor-like lesion
Eventually ossifies and disappears
Asymptomatic
Multiple lesions associated with neurofibromatosis

Epidemiology

2 to 20-year age group
Males and females affected

Location

Femur
Tibia
Fibula

Radiographic Features

Metaphyseal
Eccentric cortical geographic lucency
Long axis of lesion parallels long axis of the long bone
Endosteal scalloping
Sclerotic border

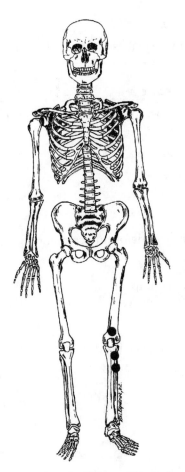

Figure 7-21 Skeletal Distribution of Fibroxanthoma. *Source:* Copyright © 1993 by Kiki Kilpatrick, D.C.

Differential Diagnosis

Classic appearance makes differential diagnosis relatively simple

7.20 Freiberg's Disease

Avascular necrosis of the second or third metatarsal distal epiphysis

Category

Avascular necrosis

General

Painful
Residual mushroom deformity common

Epidemiology

10 to 15-year age group
Females more than males

Location

Second/third metatarsal head

Radiographic Features

Sclerosis
Irregularity
Fragmentation
Flattening

Differential Diagnosis

Trauma

7.21 Giant Cell Tumor (Figures 7-22 and 7-23)

A quasimalignant skeletal neoplasm containing mainly osteoclasts; also known as an osteoclastoma

Category

Tumor/tumor-like (benign, malignant)

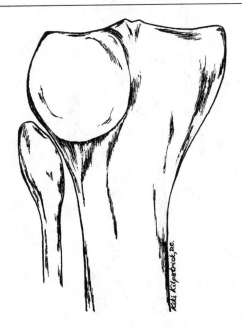

Figure 7-22 Giant Cell Tumor of the Proximal Tibia. *Source:* Copyright © 1993 by Kiki Kilpatrick, D.C.

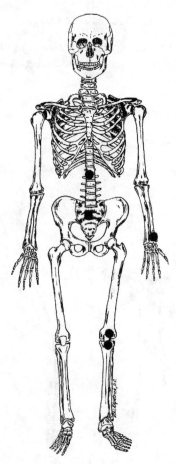

Figure 7-23 Skeletal Distribution of Giant Cell Tumor. *Source:* Copyright ©
1993 by Kiki Kilpatrick, D.C.

General

Benign and malignant forms
Difficult to differentiate benign from malignant forms
    radiographically

Epidemiology

20 to 40-year age group
Male to female 1:1

Location

Distal radius
Tibia
Femur
Spine
Sacrum

Radiographic Features

Metaphyseal
Subarticular
Eccentric
Geographic lucency
Expansile
+/– Cortical disruption
+/– Soft tissue mass

Differential Diagnosis

Aneurysmal bone cyst (younger age group, not
    subarticular)

7.22 Gout (Figure 7-24)

Multisystem disorder characterized by deposition of sodium urate crystals, most commonly in joints and kidneys

Category

Arthritides (crystal deposition arthropathy)

General

Associated with renal calculi
Associated with high purine diet

Laboratory

Elevated serum uric acid (not diagnostic)

Epidemiology

Age older than 40 years
Male to female 20:1

Location

First metatarsophalangeal joint
Elbow
Wrist
Knee
Shoulder
Hip

Radiographic Features

Periarticular tophi with calcification (50%)

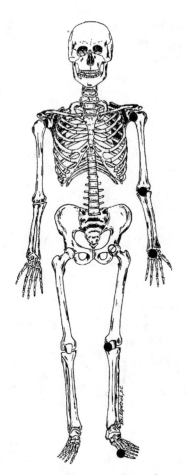

Figure 7-24 Skeletal Distribution of Gouty Arthritis. *Source:* Copyright © 1993 by Kiki Kilpatrick, D.C.

Erosions away from joint line with "overhanging edges"
Preservation of joint space
Chondrocalcinosis
No periarticular osteopenia

Differential Diagnosis

Rheumatoid arthritis (periarticular osteopenia, loss of joint
  space, no tophi)
Calcium pyrophosphate deposition disease (lack of large
  erosions/tophi)

7.23 Hemangioma (Figures 7-25 and 7-26)

Benign skeletal neoplasm characterized by anastamosing
vascular channels

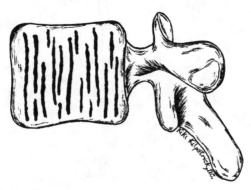

Figure 7-25 Vertebral Hemangioma. *Source:* Copyright © 1993 by Kiki
Kilpatrick, D.C.

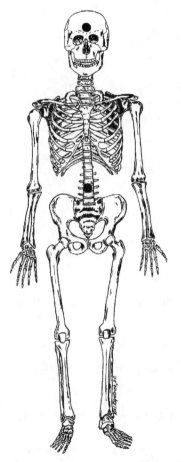

Figure 7-26 Skeletal Distribution of Hemangioma. *Source:* Copyright © 1993 by Kiki Kilpatrick, D.C.

Category

Tumor/tumor-like (benign)

General

Most common benign tumor of the spine
Two types: cavernous, capillary
Vertebral collapse unusual

Epidemiology

10 to 50-year age group
Female to male 2:1

Location

Spine
Skull

Radiographic Features

Striations within bone (vertebra = vertical, skull = radiating)
Lucent

Differential Diagnosis

Osteoporosis in spine (multiple levels)

7.24 Hemophilic Arthropathy (Figure 7-27)

X-linked abnormality of, most commonly, factor VIII or factor IX with resultant multisystem involvement, including the joints, secondary to bleeding

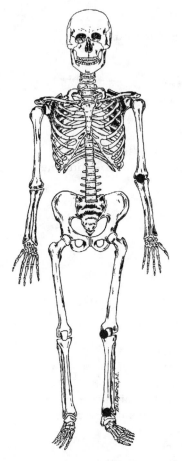

Figure 7-27 Skeletal Distribution of Hemophilic Arthropathy. *Source:* Copyright © 1993 by Kiki Kilpatrick, D.C.

Category

Arthritides (miscellaneous)

General

Pseudotumors also possible
Mimics infection clinically

Laboratory

Absent serum factor VIII/IX
Abnormal partial thromboplastin time

Epidemiology

Males only

Location

Knees
Ankles
Elbows

Radiographic Features

Opaque joint effusion
Bony enlargement
Loss of joint space
Subchondral cyst formation
Superimposed degenerative joint disease
Periarticular osteopenia
Squaring of patella
Widened intercondylar notch
Tibiotalar slant

Differential Diagnosis

Degenerative joint disease (no osteopenia, no joint effusion)

7.25 Hodgkin's Disease (Figure 7-28)

Malignant neoplasm of lymph nodes commonly secondarily affecting the skeleton

Category

Tumor/tumor-like (malignant)

General

Primary tumor of lymph nodes
Metastasizes to skeleton

Laboratory

Elevated polymorphonuclear cell count
Lymphocytopenia
Elevated alkaline phosphatase levels with skeletal involvement

Epidemiology

15 to 30-year age group

Location

Spine
Pelvis
Femur
Ribs
Skull

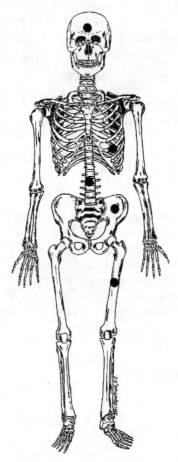

Figure 7-28 Skeletal Distribution of Hodgkin's Disease. *Source:* Copyright © 1993 by Kiki Kilpatrick, D.C.

Radiographic Features

Can be lytic, sclerotic, or mixed
Solitary sclerotic vertebra (ivory vertebra)
Anterior vertebral scalloping

Differential Diagnosis

Most malignant neoplasms

7.26 Hyperparathyroidism (Figure 7-29)

Abnormal production of parathyroid hormone with multisystem involvement

Category

Metabolic/endocrine

General

Two forms: primary, secondary to renal disease

Laboratory

Elevated serum calcium
Decreased serum phosphorus levels (suggests primary hyperparathyroidism)
Abnormalities associated with renal disease

Epidemiology

30 to 50-year age group
Female to male 3:1

Location

Hands
Sacroiliac joints

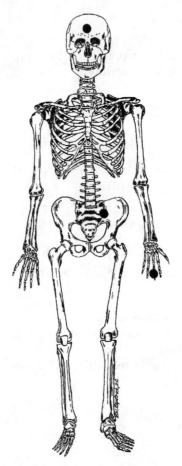

Figure 7-29 Skeletal Distribution of Hyperparathyroidism. *Source:* Copyright © 1993 by Kiki Kilpatrick, D.C.

Skull
Long bones (brown tumors)

Radiographic Features

Subperiosteal bone resorption
Radial aspects of middle phalanges of hands
Sacroiliac joints
Insertion of anconeus muscle
Vascular calcification in hands
Osteopenia (skull)
Brown tumors

Differential Diagnosis

Vascular calcification, diabetes mellitus
Brown tumor, giant cell tumor (lack of laboratory findings)

7.27 Hypertrophic Osteoarthropathy (Figure 7-30)

Periosteal new bone formation secondary to some other disease

Category

Arthritides (miscellaneous)

General

Associated with
Pulmonary disease
Gastrointestinal disease
Hepatic disease
Arteriovenous shunts in congenital cardiac disease

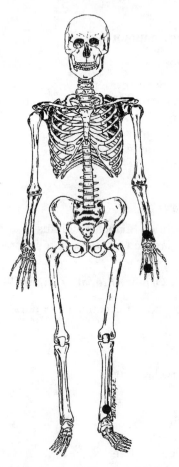

Figure 7-30 Skeletal Distribution of Hypertrophic Osteoarthropathy. *Source:* Copyright © 1993 by Kiki Kilpatrick, D.C.

Clubbing of digits also seen
Polyarthralgia also seen

Epidemiology

Dependent on etiology

Location

Tibia
Fibula
Radius
Ulna
Phalanges
Femur

Radiographic Features

Diametaphyseal
Periosteal reaction
Acral soft tissue swelling

Differential Diagnosis

Any cause of periosteal reaction

7.28 Juvenile Chronic Arthritis (Figure 7-31)

Inflammatory multisystem connective tissue disorder
with predilection for the joints

Category

Arthritides (inflammatory)

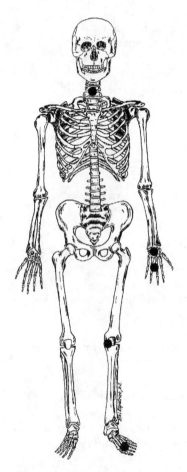

Figure 7-31 Skeletal Distribution of Juvenile Chronic Arthritis. *Source:* Copyright © 1993 by Kiki Kilpatrick, D.C.

General

Many types
Systemic onset (Still's disease)
Polyarticular onset
Oligoarticular/monarticular onset
Seropositive juvenile onset adult rheumatoid arthritis
Juvenile ankylosing spondylitis
Juvenile psoriatic arthritis
Juvenile enteropathic arthritis

Laboratory

Dependent on form of arthritis

Epidemiology

1 to 15-year age group
Females more than males

Location

Wrist
Hands
Feet
Cervical spine
Knee

Radiographic Features

Joint effusion
Periarticular osteopenia
Accelerated bone growth
Premature fusion of epiphyses

Periosteal reaction
Atlantoaxial instability
Osseous fusion

7.29 Kienböck's Disease

Avascular necrosis of the lunate

Category

Avascular necrosis

General

Associated with negative ulnar variance

Location

Wrist

Radiographic Features

Sclerosis
Fragmentation
Cyst formation
Flattening

Differential Diagnosis

Trauma

7.30 Köhler's Disease

Avascular necrosis of the tarsal navicular

Category

Avascular necrosis

General

Can be bilateral

Location

Foot

Radiographic Features

Sclerosis
Fragmentation
Cyst formation
Flattening

Differential Diagnosis

Trauma

7.31 Legg-Calvé-Perthes Disease

Avascular necrosis of the femoral capital epiphysis

Category

Avascular necrosis

General

Often bilateral
Thought to be post-traumatic

Epidemiology

3 to 8-year age group

Females more than males
African-Americans affected more commonly

Location

Femoral capital epiphysis

Radiographic Features

Sclerosis (snow cap sign)
Fragmentation
Subchondral fracture (crescent sign)
Irregularity
Joint effusion
Hypoplastic femoral capital epiphysis
Residual "mushroom" deformity

7.32 Leukemia (Figure 7-32)

Malignant neoplasm of white blood cells (WBC) with multiorgan involvement, including bone

Category

Tumor (malignant)

General

In children, almost always acute lymphoblastic leukemia
In adults, commonly chronic lymphocytic leukemia
Hepatosplenomegaly
Fever common
Skeletal changes in 50%

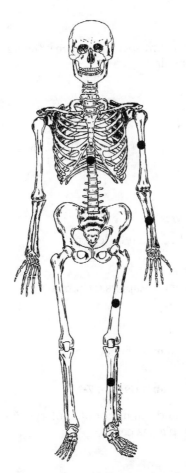

Figure 7-32 Skeletal Distribution of Changes Associated with Leukemia.
Source: Copyright © 1993 by Kiki Kilpatrick, D.C.

Laboratory

Elevated WBC count specific to type of leukemia
Thrombocytopenia
Anemia

Epidemiology

Any age group

Location

Long bones
Spine

Radiographic Features

Multiple punched-out lytic lesions
Diffuse osteopenia
Periosteal reaction
Transverse lucent metaphyseal bands
Vertebral collapse

Differential Diagnosis

Any lytic skeletal malignancy

7.33 Multiple Myeloma (Figure 7-33)

Malignant round cell tumor of adults characterized by
proliferation of plasma cells

Category

Tumor/tumor-like (malignant)

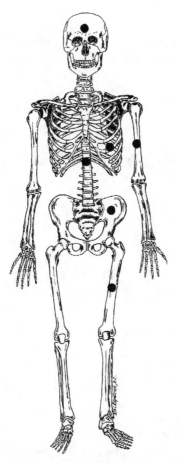

Figure 7-33 Skeletal Distribution of Multiple Myeloma. *Source:* Copyright ©
1993 by Kiki Kilpatrick, D.C.

General

Most common primary skeletal malignancy
Two major types: plasmacytoma, myelomatosis

Laboratory

Anemia
Hypercalcemia
Proteinuria
Abnormal serum protein electrophoresis

Epidemiology

Age older than 40 years
Male to female 2:1

Location

Spine
Pelvis
Skull
Ribs
Long bones

Radiographic Features

Myelomatosis
    Diffuse osteopenia
    Multiple collapsed vertebra
    Punched-out lesions in skull/long bones
Plasmacytoma
    Solitary expansile lucency

Differential Diagnosis

Osteoporosis (no pathologic collapse, more common in females)

7.34 Neurofibromatosis (Figure 7-34)

Hereditary multisystem disorder characterized by the formation of benign neural tumors and bone dysplasia

Category

Dysplasia

General

Two main types: peripheral, central
Minimal malignant potential

Epidemiology

Hereditary

Location

Skull
Spine
Long bones

Radiographic Features

Scoliosis
Enlarged dumbbell-shaped neural foramina
Posterior scalloping of vertebrae
Absent sphenoid wing

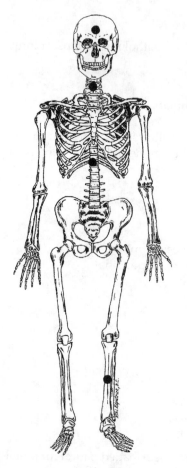

Figure 7-34 Skeletal Distribution of Neurofibromatosis. *Source:* Copyright © 1993 by Kiki Kilpatrick, D.C.

Asterion defect
Intracranial meningiomas
Anterior bowing of tibia
Pseudoarthrosis
Overtubulation of long bones

7.35 Neuropathic Arthropathy (Figure 7-35)

Aggressive destructive arthropathy secondary to lack of joint proprioception

Category

Arthritides (neuropathic arthropathy)

General

Associated with
Syringomyelia
Tertiary syphilis
Diabetes mellitus (m.c.)
Congenital insensitivity to pain
Spinal cord tumors
Meningiomyelocele
Two types: hypertrophic, atrophic
"Degenerative joint disease with an attitude"

Laboratory

Abnormalities dependent on associated disease

Epidemiology

Dependent on etiology

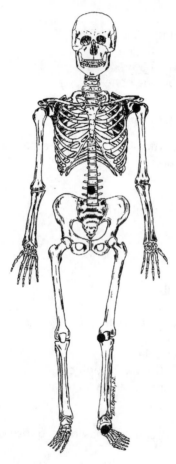

Figure 7-35 Skeletal Distribution of Neuropathic Arthropathy. *Source:* Copyright © 1993 by Kiki Kilpatrick, D.C.

Location

   Upper extremity—syringomyelia
   Spine, feet—diabetes mellitus
   Lumbar spine, knees—tertiary syphilis

Radiographic Features

   Destruction of the joint
   Debris within the joint
   Opaque joint effusion
   Sclerosis of bone
   Dislocation
   Disorganization of the joint
   Large osteophytes
   Resorption of bone (atrophic type)

Differential Diagnosis

   Relatively classic appearance

7.36 Ochronosis (Figure 7-36)

   Deposition of hemogentisic acid in connective tissue
secondary to lack of homogentisic acid oxidase

Category

   Arthritides (miscellaneous)

General

   Black pigment deposits in soft tissues
   Gray sclera

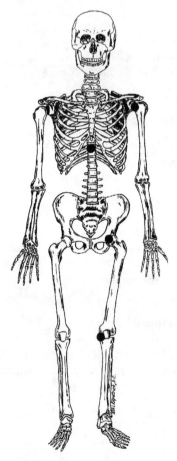

Figure 7-36 Skeletal Distribution of the Changes Associated with Ochronosis.
Source: Copyright © 1993 by Kiki Kilpatrick, D.C.

Blue-colored nasal and auricular cartilage
Also known as alkaptonuria

Laboratory

Black urine

Epidemiology

Older than age 10 years
Male to female 2:1

Location

Spine
Shoulder
Hip
Knee

Radiographic Features

Disc calcification
Precocious degenerative joint disease
Vertebral osteopenia
Multiple vacuum phenomena
Periarticular calcifications

Differential Diagnosis

Degenerative joint disease (clinical findings, age)

7.37 Osteoblastoma (Figure 7-37)

Uncommon primary benign bone tumor of osteoblastic origin with malignant potential

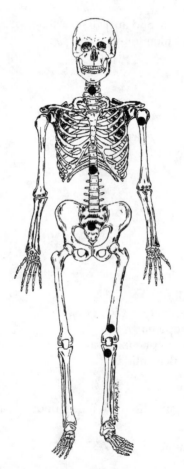

Figure 7-37 Skeletal Distribution of Osteoblastoma. *Source:* Copyright © 1993 by Kiki Kilpatrick, D.C.

Category

Tumor/tumor-like (benign)

General

Associated with a painful scoliosis

Epidemiology

5 to 30-year age group
Male to female 2:1

Location

Spine
Sacrum
Femur
Tibia
Humerus

Radiographic Features

Diametaphyseal
Neural arch of spine
Lucent nidus greater than 2 cm
Geographic
Sclerotic or lucent
Often expansile
Stippled calcification

Differential Diagnosis

Osteosarcoma (periosteal reaction)
Chondrosarcoma (periosteal reaction)

Osteoid osteoma (nidus size)
Brodie's abscess (history of infection, fever)

7.38 Osteochondroma (Figures 7-38 and 7-39)

Benign exostosis of bone with a cartilaginous cap secondary to displacement of an abnormal rest of cartilage

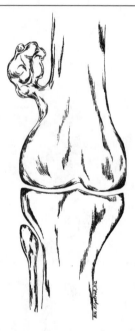

Figure 7-38 Pedunculated Osteochondroma of the Distal Femur. *Source:* Copyright © 1993 by Kiki Kilpatrick, D.C.

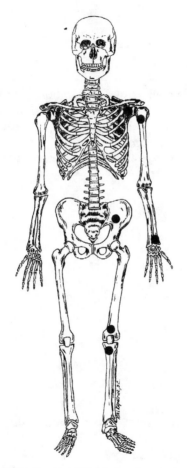

Figure 7-39 Skeletal Distribution of Osteochondroma. *Source:* Copyright © 1993 by Kiki Kilpatrick, D.C.

Category

Tumor/tumor-like (benign)

General

Can undergo malignant degeneration
Adventitious bursa may form over cartilage cap
Multiple tumors—hereditary multiple exostosis (higher
incidence of malignancy)
Only known benign tumor to occur secondary to radiation

Epidemiology

10 to 20-year age group
Males more than females

Location

Tibia
Femur
Radius
Humerus
Pelvis
Scapula

Radiographic Features

Metaphyseal
Eccentric bony outgrowth contiguous with cortex of host
bone
Sessile—broad-based
Pedunculated—connected to cortex by a stalk
Cartilage cap may calcify

Pedunculated form grows away from joint

Differential Diagnosis

Appearance is typical

7.39 Osteoid Osteoma (Figure 7-40)

Benign tumor of unknown etiology with highly vascular central nidus

Category

Tumor/tumor-like (benign)

General

Night pain relieved by salicylates (uncommon presentation)
Will recur if nidus is not completely removed
Painful scoliosis

Epidemiology

5 to 25-year age group
Male to female 2:1

Location

Found in most any bone

Radiographic Features

Small central lucent nidus
Central calcification (50%)
Large thick rim of sclerosis
Intense uptake on radionuclide bone scan

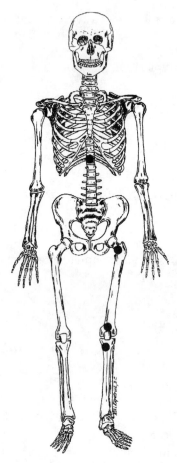

Figure 7-40 Skeletal Distribution of Osteoid Osteoma. *Source:* Copyright © 1993 by Kiki Kilpatrick, D.C.

Differential Diagnosis

Brodie's abscess (larger nidus, history of infection)
Osteoblastoma (larger nidus)
Stress fracture (no nidus, history)

7.40 Osteomyelitis (Acute) (Figure 7-41)

Acute infection of bone

Category

Infection

General

Classic signs and symptoms of infection

Laboratory

Elevated white blood cell count

Epidemiology

Children
Staphylococcus aureus is the most common causative organism

Location

Tibia
Femur
Spine

Radiographic Features

Obliteration of soft tissue fascial planes
Osseous changes not visible for 7 to 10 days

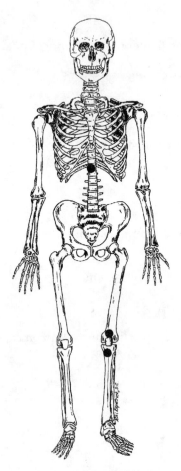

Figure 7-41 Skeletal Distribution of Osteomyelitis. *Source:* Copyright © 1993 by Kiki Kilpatrick, D.C.

Moth-eaten to permeative bone destruction
Periosteal reaction (laminated most commonly)
Sequestration of dead bone
Involucrum formation

Differential Diagnosis

Ewing's sarcoma (differentiation is difficult)

7.41 Osteosarcoma (Figure 7-42)

Primary skeletal malignancy of osteoid origin

Category

Tumor/tumor-like (malignant)

General

Second most common primary skeletal malignancy
Many forms including
    Classic central
    Telangiectatic osteosarcoma
    Postradiation osteosarcoma
    Secondary osteosarcoma
    Periosteal osteosarcoma
    Parosteal osteosarcoma
    Multifocal osteosarcoma

Epidemiology (Central Form)

10 to 25-year age group
Male to female 1.5:1

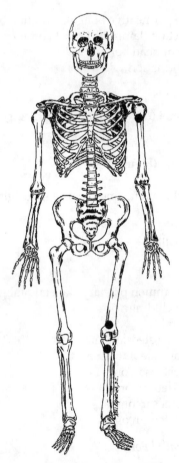

Figure 7-42 Skeletal Distribution of Osteosarcoma. *Source:* Copyright © 1993 by Kiki Kilpatrick, D.C.

Location (Central Form)

Femur
Tibia
Humerus

Radiographic Features (Central Form)

Large osteoblastic lesion
Poorly defined
Spiculated periosteal reaction
Ossified soft tissue mass

Differential Diagnosis

Radiographic presentation is classic

7.42 Paget's Disease (Figure 7-43)

Chronic inflammatory skeletal disease of probable viral etiology

Category

Miscellaneous

General

Also known as osteitis deformans
Patient may present with enlarging hat size for unknown reasons
Associated with basilar invagination and spinal canal stenosis
May undergo sarcomatous malignant degeneration

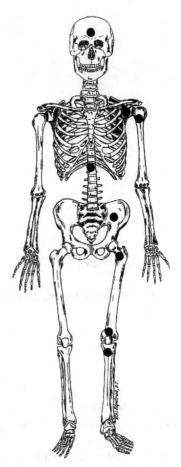

Figure 7-43 Skeletal Distribution of Paget's Disease of Bone. *Source*: Copyright © 1993 by Kiki Kilpatrick, D.C.

Three stages
  Lytic
  Blastic
  Mixed

Epidemiology

  40 to 60-year age group
  Male to female 2:1

Location

  Skull
  Pelvis
  Spine
  Tibia
  Femur
  Humerus
  Scapula

Radiographic Features

  Focal areas of bone lysis (e.g., skull—osteoporosis
    circumscripta)
  Bony enlargement
  Trabecular accentuation
  Thickened cortex

Differential Diagnosis

  Fibrous dysplasia (differentiation can be difficult)

7.43 Panner's Disease

Avascular necrosis of the capitullum

Category

Avascular necrosis

General

Chronic elbow pain
May lead to early degenerative joint disease

Epidemiology

Adolescents

Location

Capitullum

Radiographic Features

Sclerosis
Irregularity
Fragmentation
Flattening

Differential Diagnosis

Trauma

7.44 Primary Lymphoma of Bone (Figure 7-44)

Primary round cell malignancy of bone, previously known as reticulum cell sarcoma

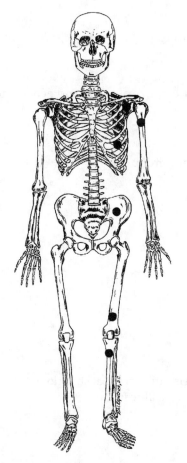

Figure 7-44 Skeletal Distribution of Primary Lymphoma of Bone. *Source:*
Copyright © 1993 by Kiki Kilpatrick, D.C.

Category

Tumor/tumor-like (malignant)

General

Great difference in size of lesion and general health of patient

Epidemiology

30 to 50-year age group
Male to female 2:1

Location

Femur
Tibia
Humerus
Pelvis
Scapula
Ribs

Radiographic Features

Diaphyseal
Ill-defined permeative bone destruction
Laminated periosteal reaction
Soft tissue mass

Differential Diagnosis

Osteomyelitis
Osteosarcoma

7.45 Progressive Systemic Sclerosis

Inflammatory connective tissue disease causing sclerosis of small arteries and its sequelae in multiple organ systems

Category

Arthritides (connective tissue arthropathy)
Also known as scleroderma

Laboratory

Positive rheumatoid factor in one-third of patients
Positive antinuclear antibody (90%)

General

Associated with
    Soft tissue calcification
    Raynaud's phenomenon
    Esophageal dysmotility
    Telangiectasia

Epidemiology

30 to 50-year age group
Females more than males

Location

Hands

Radiographic Features

Resorption of terminal tufts of fingers
Soft tissue calcification
No periarticular osteopenia

7.46 Reiter's Syndrome (Figure 7-45)

Inflammatory spinal arthropathy associated with a classic clinical triad

Category

Arthritides (seronegative spondyloarthropathy)

General

Triad—arthritis, conjunctivitis, urethritis
Also associated with
  Balanitis circinata
  Keratoderma blennorrhagicum
  Vaginitis
History of sexually transmitted disease common
Positive histocompatibility locus antigen-B27 in most
  patients

Laboratory

Positive histocompatibility locus antigen-B27
Elevated erythrocyte sedimentation rate

Epidemiology

Young males

Location

Spine
Knees
Ankles
Feet

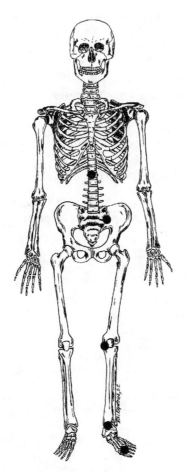

Figure 7-45 Skeletal Distribution of Reiter's Syndrome. *Source:* Copyright © 1993 by Kiki Kilpatrick, D.C.

Radiographic Features

Hazy erosions of bone
Asymmetric sacroiliitis
Parasyndesmophytes
Fluffy periosteal new bone formation

Differential Diagnosis

Other seronegative spondyloarthropathies (history)

7.47 Rheumatoid Arthritis (Figure 7-46)

Inflammatory connective tissue disease of unknown etiology with polyarthropathy as its primary feature

Category

Arthritides (inflammatory)

General

Bilaterally symmetric disease
Atlantoaxial subluxation possible
Basilar invagination possible

Laboratory

Positive rheumatoid factor
Positive histocompatibility locus antigen-DR4
Elevated erythrocyte sedimentation rate

Epidemiology

30 to 60-year age group
Female to male 3:1

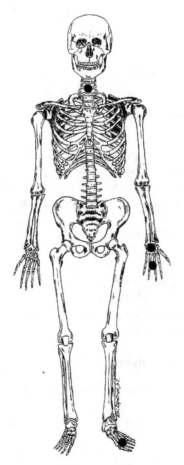

Figure 7-46 Skeletal Distribution of Rheumatoid Arthritis. *Source:* Copyright ©
1993 by Kiki Kilpatrick, D.C.

Location

Hands
Feet
Cervical spine
Wrists

Radiographic Features

Fusiform soft tissue swelling
Concentric loss of joint space
Periarticular osteopenia
Marginal erosions of bone
Fibrous ankylosis of joints (except bony ankylosis in carpus
    and tarsus)
Subchondral cyst formation

Differential Diagnosis

Seronegative spondyloarthropathies (bony ankylosis,
    lumbar spine involvement)
Systemic lupus erythematosus (no erosions, no joint de-
    struction until late)

7.48 Scheuermann's Disease

Vertebral epiphysitis secondary to repetitive trauma

Category

Trauma

General

Clinical kyphosis

Usually seen in active patients
Self-resolving

Epidemiology

Adolescents

Location

Thoracolumbar spine

Radiographic Features

Multiple Schmorl's nodes
Kyphosis
Loss of anterior vertebral body height

7.49 Sickle Cell Anemia (Figure 7-47)

Hereditary abnormality of hemoglobin in red blood cells
that results in sickling of the cells and its multiorgan
sequelae

Category

Hematologic

General

Ischemia
Infarction
Infection

Laboratory

Anemia
Presence of sickled cells on peripheral smear

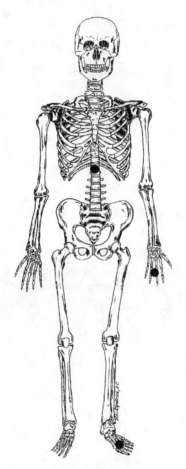

Figure 7-47 Skeletal Distribution of the Changes Associated with Sickle Cell Anemia. *Source:* Copyright © 1993 by Kiki Kilpatrick, D.C.

Epidemiology

African-American patients

Location

Hands
Feet
Spine

Radiographic Features

Avascular necrosis of bone
Medullary bone infarcts
Osteomyelitis (*Salmonella* m.c.)

Differential Diagnosis

Other anemias (less osseous findings)

7.50 Simple Bone Cyst (Figures 7-48 and 7-49)

Benign tumor-like cyst of bone

Category

Tumor/tumor-like (benign)

General

Pathologic fracture common
Asymptomatic unless fractured

Epidemiology

5 to 20-year age group
Male to female 2:1

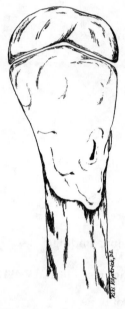

Figure 7-48 Simple Bone Cyst with a "Fallen Fragment." *Source:* Copyright © 1993 by Kiki Kilpatrick, D.C.

Location

Humerus
Femur
Calcaneus

Radiographic Features

Geographic lucency
Expansile

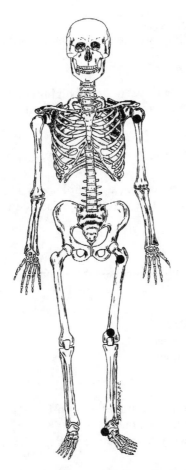

Figure 7-49 Skeletal Distribution of Simple Bone Cysts. *Source*: Copyright ©
1993 by Kiki Kilpatrick, D.C.

Central metaphysis
Migrates to diaphysis with increasing age

Differential Diagnosis

Aneurysmal bone cyst (painful, highly expansile, eccentric)
Giant cell tumor (age, painful, subarticular)

7.51 Systemic Lupus Erythematosus (Figure 7-50)

Connective tissue disease of unknown etiology resulting in microvasculopathy and its sequelae in multiple organ systems

Category

Arthritides (connective tissue arthropathy)

General

Butterfly malar rash
Pulmonary disease
Hepatosplenomegaly

Laboratory

Positive antinuclear antibodies/anti-DNA antibodies
Negative rheumatoid factor
Positive lupus erythematosus cell preparation

Epidemiology

Young females

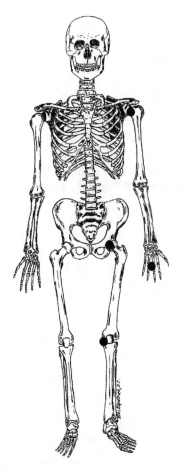

Figure 7-50 Skeletal Distribution of Systemic Lupus Erythematosus. *Source:* Copyright © 1993 by Kiki Kilpatrick, D.C.

Location

Hands
Knee
Hip
Shoulder

Radiographic Features

Periarticular osteopenia
Soft tissue swelling
Reversible subluxation of the joints of the hands
Avascular necrosis of the femoral head

Differential Diagnosis

Rheumatoid arthritis (erosions)

Bibliography

NEUROMUSCULAR DISEASES

Chapman S., Nakielny R. 1990. *Aids to radiological differential diagnosis*. Philadelphia: Bailliere Tindall.

Dejong R. 1979. *The neurologic examination*. New York: Harper & Row.

Friedman A., Wilkins R. 1984. *Neurosurgical management for the house officer*. Baltimore: Williams & Wilkins.

Goldberg S. 1990. *Clinical neuroanatomy made ridiculously simple*. Miami: Medmaster.

Juhl J., Crummy A., eds. 1987. *Essentials of radiologic imaging*. Philadelphia: JB Lippincott.

Lawrence D. 1990. *Fundamentals of chiropractic diagnosis and management*. Baltimore: Williams & Wilkins.

Mumenthaler M. 1983. *Neurology: A textbook for physicians and students with 185 self-testing questions*. New York: Theime-Stratton.

Osborn A. 1991. *Handbook of neuroradiology*. St. Louis: Mosby.

Salter R. 1983. *Textbook of disorders and injuries of the musculo-skeletal system*. Baltimore: Williams & Wilkins.

Taveras J., Ferucci J. 1987. *Radiology, diagnosis-imaging-intervention*. Philadelphia: JB Lippincott.

Thurston S. 1987. *The little black book of neurology*. Chicago: Yearbook Medical Publishers.

Wyatt L. 1992. *Handbook of clinical chiropractic*. Gaithersburg, Maryland: Aspen Publishers.

SKELETAL DISEASES

Forrester D., Brown J., Nesson J. 1978. *The radiology of joint disease*. Philadelphia: WB Saunders.

Jaeger S., Pate D. 1990. *Case studies in chiropractic radiology*. Gaithersburg, Maryland: Aspen Publishers.

Juhl J., Crummy A., eds. 1987. *Essentials of radiologic imaging*. Philadelphia: JB Lippincott.

Resnick D., Niwayama G. 1988. *Diagnosis of bone and joint disorders*. Philadelphia: WB Saunders.

Yochum T., Rowe L. 1987. *Essentials of skeletal radiology*. Baltimore: Williams & Wilkins.

Index